W9-BGC-147

ELSEVIER

1600 John F. Kennedy Boulevard • Suite 1800 • Philadelphia, Pennsylvania, 19103-2899

http://www.pet.theclinics.com

PET CLINICS Volume 9, Number 3
July 2014 ISSN 1556-8598, ISBN-13: 978-0-323-31168-7

Editor: John Vassallo (j.vassallo@elsevier.com)
Developmental Editor: Susan Showalter

PET Clinics (ISSN 1556-8598) is published quarterly by Elsevier Inc., 360 Park Avenue South, New York, NY 10010-1710. Months of issue are January, April, July, and October. Periodicals postage paid at New York, NY, and additional mailing offices. Subscription prices per year are $225.00 (US individuals), $327.00 (US institutions), $115.00 (US students), $255.00 (Canadian individuals), $369.00 (Canadian institutions), $140.00 (Canadian students), $275.00 (foreign individuals), $369.00 (foreign institutions), and $140.00 (foreign students). To receive student and resident rate, orders must be accompanied by name of affiliated institution, date of term, and the signature of program/residency coordinator on institution letterhead. Orders will be billed at individual rate until proof of status is received. Foreign air speed delivery is included in all Clinics subscription prices. All prices are subject to change without notice. POSTMASTER: Send address changes to PET Clinics, Elsevier Health Sciences Division, Subscription Customer Service, 3251 Riverport Lane, Maryland Heights, MO 63043. **Customer Service: 1-800-654-2452 (U.S. and Canada); 314-447-8871 (outside U.S. and Canada). Fax: 314-447-8029. E-mail: journalscustomerservice-usa@elsevier.com (for print support); journalsonlinesupport-usa@elsevier.com (for online support).**

Reprints. For copies of 100 or more of articles in this publication, please contact the Commercial Reprints Department, Elsevier Inc., 360 Park Avenue South, New York, NY 10010-1710. Tel.: 212-633-3874; Fax: 212-633-3820; E-mail: reprints@elsevier.com.

Printed in the United States of America.

Contributors

CONSULTING EDITOR

ABASS ALAVI, MD, PhD (Hon), Dsc (Hon)
Professor of Radiology, Division of Nuclear Medicine, Department of Radiology, University of Pennsylvania School of Medicine, Hospital of the University of Pennsylvania, Philadelphia, Pennsylvania

EDITORS

CHUN K. KIM, MD
Associate Professor of Radiology, Harvard Medical School; Clinical Director, Division of Nuclear Medicine and Molecular Imaging, Department of Radiology, Brigham and Women's Hospital, Boston, Massachusetts

MOHSEN BEHESHTI, MD, FASNC, FEBNM
Head, PET-CT Center LINZ, Associate Professor in Nuclear Medicine, Department of Nuclear Medicine and Endocrinology, St Vincent's Hospital, Linz, Austria

AUTHORS

ABASS ALAVI, MD, PhD (Hon), Dsc (Hon)
Professor of Radiology, Division of Nuclear Medicine, Department of Radiology, University of Pennsylvania School of Medicine, Hospital of the University of Pennsylvania, Philadelphia, Pennsylvania

VALENTINA AMBROSINI, MD, PhD
Assistant Professor, Nuclear Medicine, S.Orsola-Malpighi University Hospital, Bologna, Italy

LIDIJA ANTUNOVIC, MD
Nuclear Medicine Department, Humanitas Clinical and Research Institute, Rozzano, Milan, Italy

MOHSEN BEHESHTI, MD, FASNC, FEBNM
Head, PET-CT Center LINZ, Associate Professor in Nuclear Medicine, Department of Nuclear Medicine and Endocrinology, St Vincent's Hospital, Linz, Austria

JAMSHED B. BOMANJI, MD, MBBS, PhD, FRCR, FRCP
Head of Clinical Department, Institute of Nuclear Medicine, T5 University College London Hospital, London, United Kingdom

ANDREAS K. BUCK, MD
Department of Nuclear Medicine, Universitätsklinikum Würzburg, Würzburg, Germany

ARTURO CHITI, MD
Nuclear Medicine Department, Humanitas Clinical and Research Institute, Rozzano, Milan, Italy

SOTIRIOS CHONDROGIANNIS, MD
Department of Nuclear Medicine, PET/CT Centre, Santa Maria della Misericordia Hospital, Rovigo, Italy

EINAT EVEN-SAPIR, MD, PhD
Head, Department of Nuclear Medicine,
Tel-Aviv Sourasky Medical Center, Sackler
Faculty of Medicine, Tel-Aviv University,
Tel-Aviv, Israel

STEFANO FANTI, MD
Associate Professor, Nuclear Medicine,
S.Orsola-Malpighi University Hospital,
Bologna, Italy

FREDERICK D. GRANT, MD
Division of Nuclear Medicine and Molecular
Imaging, Department of Radiology,
Boston Children's Hospital; Assistant
Professor in Radiology, Harvard Medical
School; Training Program Director, Joint
Program in Nuclear Medicine, Department
of Radiology, Harvard Medical School,
Boston, Massachusetts

ATHAR HAROON, FRCR
Consultant Nuclear Medicine, University
College London Hospital, London,
United Kingdom

KEN HERRMANN, MD
Department of Nuclear Medicine,
Universitätsklinikum Würzburg, Würzburg,
Germany

GEORGIOS KARANIKAS, MD
Division of Nuclear Medicine, PET-PET/CT,
Department of Biomedical Imaging and
Image-Guided Therapy, Medical University
of Vienna, Vienna, Austria

CHUN K. KIM, MD
Associate Professor of Radiology,
Harvard Medical School; Clinical Director,
Division of Nuclear Medicine and Molecular
Imaging, Department of Radiology, Brigham
and Women's Hospital, Boston,
Massachusetts

WERNER LANGSTEGER, MD, FACE
Professor and Chairman, PET-CT Center
LINZ, Department of Nuclear Medicine and
Endocrinology, St Vincent's Hospital, Linz,
Austria

MARIA CRISTINA MARZOLA, MD
Department of Nuclear Medicine, PET/CT
Centre, Santa Maria della Misericordia
Hospital, Rovigo, Italy

CRISTINA NANNI, MD
Nuclear Medicine, S.Orsola-Malpighi
University Hospital, Bologna, Italy

LORENZO NARDO, MD
Department of Radiology and Biomedical
Imaging, University of California,
San Francisco, California; Department
of Radiology, Brescia, Italy

MIGUEL HERNANDEZ PAMPALONI, MD, PhD
Chief, Nuclear Medicine, Department of
Radiology and Biomedical Imaging, University
of California, San Francisco, California

MARCELLO RODARI, MD
Nuclear Medicine Department, Humanitas
Clinical and Research Institute, Rozzano,
Milan, Italy

PIETRO ROSSI, MS
Nuclear Medicine Department, Humanitas
Clinical and Research Institute, Rozzano,
Milan, Italy

DOMENICO RUBELLO, MD
Director, Department of Nuclear Medicine,
PET/CT Centre, Santa Maria della Misericordia
Hospital, Rovigo, Italy

TARUN SINGHAL, MD
Division of Nuclear Medicine and Molecular
Imaging, Department of Radiology, Brigham
and Women's Hospital, Harvard Medical
School, Boston, Massachusetts

Contents

Preface: PET Tracers Beyond FDG: Normal Variations and Benign Findings   xi

Chun K. Kim and Mohsen Beheshti

Standardization and Quantification in PET/CT Imaging: Tracers Beyond FDG   259

Lidija Antunovic, Marcello Rodari, Pietro Rossi, and Arturo Chiti

Standardized procedures are fundamental to ensure reproducibility of medical actions. Diagnostic imaging is required to be standard as well, particularly when it has to be used as a biomarker in clinical trials. Several standard procedures and guidelines are available for the use of PET/CT with [18F]Fluorodeoxyglucose in oncology, because of the high number of procedures performed worldwide. On the other hand, standardized procedures are still lacking for PET/CT using other radiopharmaceuticals.

Brain: Positron Emission Tomography Tracers Beyond [18F]Fluorodeoxyglucose   267

Tarun Singhal, Abass Alavi, and Chun K. Kim

Several positron emission tomography (PET) radiopharmaceuticals beyond fluorodeoxyglucose (FDG) have been used to study the physiology and pathophysiology in neurosciences. This article provides a broad overview of some of the commonly studied radiopharmaceuticals for PET imaging in selected neurologic conditions, particularly attempting to study their clinical relevance. Future studies on the use of advanced PET imaging in delineating neural pathophysiology, drug development, and altering patient management and outcomes across the disciplines of neurosciences are needed.

18F-Fluoride PET/Computed Tomography Imaging   277

Einat Even-Sapir

Production of 18F-labeled tracers, including 18F-fluoride, has been simplified, and bone imaging using 18F-fluoride PET with computed tomography (PET/CT) is relevant once again. 18F-Fluoride PET/CT imaging should be considered for the assessment of bone abnormality in clinical practice, not only in patients with cancer but also in benign scenarios. Accumulated data on the use of 18F-fluoride indicate that this modality is highly sensitive for the detection of skeletal lesions, allowing assessment of pathophysiologic processes in normal and abnormal bone.

18F-Fluoride PET and PET/CT in Children and Young Adults   287

Frederick D. Grant

In children and young adults, 18F-fluoride PET and PET/computed tomography (CT) are used to evaluate a wide variety of benign and malignant skeletal disorders, but most studies are performed to evaluate nonmalignant conditions. One of the most common indications in children and young adults is the evaluation of back pain. 18F-fluoride PET and PET/CT also can be helpful in the assessment of children with suspected abuse. Less commonly in children, 18F-fluoride PET/CT is used to evaluate skeleton pain at other sites and to evaluate for osseous metastases.

Fluorocholine PET/Computed Tomography: Physiologic Uptake, Benign Findings, and Pitfalls   299

Mohsen Beheshti, Athar Haroon, Jamshed B. Bomanji, and Werner Langsteger

> This article addresses potential pitfalls and strengths of choline as a tracer in PET imaging. Choline acts as a precursor for the biosynthesis of phosphatidylcholine and other phospholipids. Because there is an increase in cell proliferation in cancers, the demand for phospholipids is high. This high content of phosphorylcholine in most cancers has been demonstrated with ^{31}P nuclear magnetic resonance studies, whereas normal tissues have low levels. During the past decade the use of new PET tracers, namely ^{11}C- and ^{18}F-labeled choline analogues, has been increasing. The physiologic pattern of choline-labeled radiotracer uptake and its related benign findings are reviewed.

^{18}F-DOPA PET/Computed Tomography Imaging   307

Sotirios Chondrogiannis, Maria Cristina Marzola, and Domenico Rubello

> In recent years, the radiopharmaceutical ^{18}F-DOPA has gained increasing application in the management of disorders such as neuroendocrine tumors, brain tumors, and pancreatic cell hyperplasia. Despite showing promising results, the role of ^{18}F-DOPA is not yet fully accepted, mainly because of its difficult radiosynthesis and availability. Moreover, procedures on administration activity, acquisition timing, and premedication with carbidopa are not standardized. This article presents the main clinical applications of ^{18}F-DOPA PET/computed tomography, focusing on the physiologic biodistribution of the tracer and its normal variants, and describing possible pitfalls that could lead to misinterpretations of scans in various clinical settings.

The Use of Gallium-68 Labeled Somatostatin receptors in PET/CT Imaging   323

Valentina Ambrosini, Cristina Nanni, and Stefano Fanti

> Somatostatin receptors (SSTRs) are expressed on neuroendocrine cells widely dispersed in the human body. Neuroendocrine tumors (NET) are characterized by increased SSTR expression and may virtually arise anywhere in the human body. The diagnostic flowchart of NET patients has been completely revolutionized in the past few years as a consequence of the development of new radiotracers for PET/computed tomographic imaging. In particular, 68Ga-DOTA-SSTRTs are a family of β-emitting tracers that specifically bind to SSTR and are increasingly used for the detection of NET in clinical trials in Europe.

Proliferation Imaging with ^{18}F-Fluorothymidine PET/Computed Tomography: Physiologic Uptake, Variants, and Pitfalls   331

Ken Herrmann and Andreas K. Buck

> This article gives a short introduction to the rationale of proliferation imaging with PET and the thymidine analogue 3'-deoxy-3'-[^{18}F]fluorothymidine (FLT). The physiologic distribution of FLT, clinical indications, and specific variants are presented. Potential pitfalls leading to relevant limitations of FLT PET/computed tomography are discussed.

^{11}C-Acetate PET/CT Imaging: Physiologic Uptake, Variants, and Pitfalls   339

Georgios Karanikas and Mohsen Beheshti

> ^{11}C-acetate PET is used in the assessment of various cardiologic and oncologic diseases. This article describes the physiologic uptake of ^{11}C-acetate and presents the

common benign findings in different anatomic parts of the body. Salivary glands, tonsils, thyroid, meningeal tuberculoma, meningiomas, and macroadenomas of the pituitary gland are sites of mild to moderate tracer uptake in the head and neck region. Parenchymal diseases of the lung and reactive and/or inflammatory mediastinal lymphadenopathies cause benign ^{11}C-acetate uptake in the thorax. Liver, spleen, pancreas, and rectum show an increased uptake. Urinary tract and prostate gland show faint tracer uptake.

PET/MRI Radiotracer Beyond ^{18}F-FDG   345

Miguel Hernandez Pampaloni and Lorenzo Nardo

The recent development and introduction of new hybrid imaging devices combining positron emission tomography (PET) technology with magnetic resonance imaging (MRI) opens up new perspectives in clinical molecular imaging. Combining MRI and fluorine-18 choline PET would theoretically produce valuable clinical data in a single imaging session, which can be used for staging, prognosis, and assessment of treatment response. Fluorine-18–sodium fluoride (^{18}F-NaF) is a highly sensitive PET tracer used as a marker of osteoblastic abnormalities. PET imaging with ^{68}Ga-DOTATATE or DOTATOC has demonstrated promising results for locating metastatic lesions, occasionally with superior sensitivity than whole-body MRI. L-DOPA PET adds data regarding L-DOPA metabolism, which may increase the specificity and sensibility of the study itself. Fluoromisonidazole is known to be not only a useful tracer for determining hypoxic cells but also an efficient hypoxic radiosensitizer.

Index   351

PET CLINICS

FORTHCOMING ISSUES

October 2014
Contributions of FDG to Modern Medicine, Part I
Søren Hess and Poul Flemming Høilund-Carlsen, *Editors*

January 2015
Clinical Applications of FDG, Part II
Søren Hess and Poul Flemming Høilund-Carlsen, *Editors*

April 2015
PET/CT and Patient Outcomes in Oncology, Part I
Rathan M. Subramaniam, *Editor*

RECENT ISSUES

April 2014
FDG PET/CT Imaging: Normal Variations and Benign Findings
Mohsen Beheshti and Chun K. Kim, *Editors*

January 2014
Management of Neuroendocrine Tumors
Stefano Fanti, Cristina Nanni, and Richard Baum, *Editors*

October 2013
Novel Imaging Techniques in Neurodegenerative and Movement Disorders
Rathan M. Subramaniam and Jorge R. Barrio, *Editors*

PROGRAM OBJECTIVE

The goal of the PET Clinics is to keep practicing radiologists and radiology residents up to date with current clinical practice in positron emission tomography by providing timely articles reviewing the state of the art in patient care.

TARGET AUDIENCE

Practicing radiologists, radiology residents, and other health care professionals who provide patient care utilizing radiologic findings.

LEARNING OBJECTIVES

Upon completion of this activity, participants will be able to:
1. Review 18F-flouride PET and PET/CT in all populations including children and young adults.
2. Discuss standardization and quantification in PET/CT Imaging.
3. Discuss normal variations and benign findings beyond FDG in PET/CT Imaging.

ACCREDITATION

The Elsevier Office of Continuing Medical Education (EOCME) is accredited by the Accreditation Council for Continuing Medical Education (ACCME) to provide continuing medical education for physicians.

The EOCME designates this enduring material for a maximum of 15 *AMA PRA Category 1 Credit*(s)™. Physicians should claim only the credit commensurate with the extent of their participation in the activity.

All other health care professionals requesting continuing education credit for this enduring material will be issued a certificate of participation.

DISCLOSURE OF CONFLICTS OF INTEREST

The EOCME assesses conflict of interest with its instructors, faculty, planners, and other individuals who are in a position to control the content of CME activities. All relevant conflicts of interest that are identified are thoroughly vetted by EOCME for fair balance, scientific objectivity, and patient care recommendations. EOCME is committed to providing its learners with CME activities that promote improvements or quality in healthcare and not a specific proprietary business or a commercial interest.

The planning committee, staff, authors and editors listed below have identified no financial relationships or relationships to products or devices they or their spouse/life partner have with commercial interest related to the content of this CME activity:

Abass Alavi, MD; Valentina Ambrosini, MD, PhD; Lidija Antunovic, MD; Mohsen Beheshti, MD, FEBNM, FASNC; Jamshed B. Bomanji, MD, MBBS, PhD, FRCR, FRCP; Andreas K. Buck, MD; Arturo Chiti, MD; Sotirios Chondrogiannis, MD; Einat Even-Sapir, MD, PhD; Stefano Fanti, MD; Frederick D. Grant, MD; Athar Haroon, FRCR; Kristen Helm; Ken Herrmann, MD; Brynne Hunter; Georgios Karanikas, MD; Chun K. Kim, MD; Werner Langsteger, MD, FACE; Sandy Lavery; Maria Cristina Marzola, MD; Jill McNair; Cristina Nanni, MD; Mahalakshmi Narayanan; Lorenzo Nardo, MD; Miguel Hernandez Pampaloni, MD, PhD; Marcello Rodari, MD; Pietro Rossi, MS; Domenico Rubello, MD; Tarun Singhal, MD; John Vassallo.

The planning committee, staff, authors and editors listed below have identified financial relationships or relationships to products or devices they or their spouse/life partner have with commercial interest related to the content of this CME activity:

UNAPPROVED/OFF-LABEL USE DISCLOSURE

The EOCME requires CME faculty to disclose to the participants:
1. When products or procedures being discussed are off-label, unlabelled, experimental, and/or investigational (not US Food and Drug Administration (FDA) approved); and
2. Any limitations on the information presented, such as data that are preliminary or that represent ongoing research, interim analyses, and/or unsupported opinions. Faculty may discuss information about pharmaceutical agents that is outside of FDA-approved labelling. This information is intended solely for CME and is not intended to promote off-label use of these medications. If you have any questions, contact the medical affairs department of the manufacturer for the most recent prescribing information.

TO ENROLL

To enroll in the PET Clinics Continuing Medical Education program, call customer service at 1-800-654-2452 or sign up online at http://www.theclinics.com/home/cme. The CME program is available to subscribers for an additional annual fee of USD 235.

METHOD OF PARTICIPATION

In order to claim credit, participants must complete the following:
1. Complete enrolment as indicated above.
2. Read the activity.
3. Complete the CME Test and Evaluation. Participants must achieve a score of 70% on the test. All CME Tests and Evaluations must be completed online.

CME INQUIRIES/SPECIAL NEEDS

For all CME inquiries or special needs, please contact elsevierCME@elsevier.com.

Preface

PET Tracers Beyond FDG: Normal Variations and Benign Findings

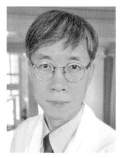
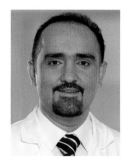

Chun K. Kim, MD   Mohsen Beheshti, MD, FASNC, FEBNM

Editors

The unique usefulness of PET lies in its ability to image the in vivo distribution and kinetics of a wide variety of biomolecules labeled with positron-emitting radioisotopes. While [F-18]-FDG has been the workhorse of PET imaging, a number of other PET radiopharmaceuticals have been studied extensively in oncologic, cardiovascular, and neurologic disorders. These agents study biologic processes and molecular targets other than those involved in glucose metabolism, such as amino acid metabolism, purine and pyrimidine metabolism, cell turnover, receptors and transporters, abnormal protein deposition, bone turnover, and others. Newer approaches toward labeling of probes, image acquisition, and analysis and "fusion" of PET imaging with MRI have added extensive enthusiasm in the field. This issue of *PET Clinics* aims to review some of the extensively studied non-FDG PET radiopharmaceuticals with regard to their potential clinical usefulness, normal variations, benign findings, and pitfalls.

The first article, by Antunovic and colleagues, emphasizes the need for, and provides an overview of, the ongoing efforts related to the standardization and quantification of non-FDG radiopharmaceuticals for PET imaging. Specific examples of [C-11] methionine and [C-11] choline are highlighted.

The second article, by Singhal and colleagues, provides an overview of non-FDG PET radiopharmaceuticals used to assess various neurologic conditions, including dementia, movement disorders, epilepsy, brain tumors, and neuroinflammation.

There is a renewed interest in [F-18] sodium fluoride bone imaging, likely due to the increasing availability of PET/CT scanners, improved logistics for the delivery of F-18-labeled radiotracers, and the higher quality images that can be acquired with PET/CT. The next two articles, written by Even-Sapir and Grant, review [F-18] sodium fluoride PET, focusing on adult and pediatric applications, respectively.

The uptake of [F-18] choline is a marker of cellular proliferation and is potentially useful in several malignancies. Along with the physiologic uptake, benign variations, and effects of various treatments, the role of [F-18] choline is the subject of discussion in the article by Beheshti and colleagus.

The article by Chondrogiannis and colleagues reviews [F-18] DOPA that was originally developed to study the integrity of the striatal dopaminergic system in the central nervous system but has additionally demonstrated efficacy for the evaluation of neuroendocrine tumors, brain tumors, and pancreatic cell hyperplasia.

Radiolabeling of somatostatin receptor ligands with the generator-produced positron emitter gallium-68 using a chelator, such as DOTA, is an example of an alternate approach to labeling PET radiopharmaceuticals and has significantly advanced the field of somatostatin receptor imaging. The various Ga-68-labeled somatostatin receptor

PET Clin 9 (2014) xi–xii
http://dx.doi.org/10.1016/j.cpet.2014.04.001

agents (DOTA-TOC, DOTA-NOC, and DOTA-TATE) are reviewed in the article by Ambrosini and colleagues.

The following article by Herrmann and Buck reviews [F-18] fluorothymidine, a marker of cellular proliferation, with potential usefulness in a large number of oncologic conditions, including in the diagnosis and assessment of treatment response.

[C-11] acetate is a biomarker for cell membrane lipid synthesis and also undergoes both catabolic and anabolic metabolism. Its use in various cardiologic and oncologic conditions and relevant variations and imaging pitfalls are reviewed in the article by Karanikas and Beheshti.

PET/MRI using non-FDG PET ligands is an exciting, synergistic technology with relevance across medical and surgical subspecialties and is the subject of the review of the final article, by Pampaloni and Nardo.

Overall, the current issue of the *PET Clinics* provides a comprehensive overview of some of the key aspects of PET imaging, with tracers beyond FDG, particularly their main clinical usefulness, normal variations, benign findings, and potential pitfalls. We hope that the readers will find this issue informative and useful, and that it will stimulate further research to enhance our understanding of pathophysiology of various diseases and to improve patient care. Finally, we would like to thank the authors for sharing their expertise and making a valuable contribution to the field.

Chun K. Kim, MD
Division of Nuclear Medicine and
Molecular Imaging
Department of Radiology
Brigham and Women's Hospital
Harvard Medical School
Boston, Massachusetts

Mohsen Beheshti, MD, FASNC, FEBNM
PET-CT Center Linz
Department of Nuclear Medicine and
Endocrinology
St. Vincent's Hospital
Linz, Austria

E-mail addresses:
ckkim@bwh.harvard.edu (C.K. Kim)
Mohsen.Beheshti@bhs.at (M. Beheshti)

Standardization and Quantification in PET/CT Imaging: Tracers Beyond FDG

Lidija Antunovic, MD, Marcello Rodari, MD, Pietro Rossi, MS, Arturo Chiti, MD*

KEYWORDS

- Positron emission tomography • Radiopharmaceuticals • Imaging • Harmonization
- Standardization • Quantification

KEY POINTS

- Standardization and harmonization of PET images are required to use the technique as an imaging biomarker in oncology.
- Standardization programs are in place mainly for fludeoxyglucose F18 studies, because this radiopharmaceutical is widely used and distributed throughout the world.
- Few initiatives are running on the standardization of PET/computed tomography procedures with non-FDG radiopharmaceuticals.
- Existing initiatives concern [68]Ga-(DOTA[0]-Phe[1]-Tyr[3]) octreotide and ^{11}C-methionine.

INTRODUCTION

Modern medicine is aiming for personalized treatment to every single patient. Although this will not be possible in the near future, molecular characteristics of the tumor and its interrelation with the host, the patient itself, can guide the use of therapies that are designed to be effective in groups of individuals.

Imaging biomarkers can play a role in identifying patient and tumors' characteristics, which are going to influence the response to the therapy and, ultimately, patient's outcome.

PET, allowing imaging of the biodistribution of radiolabeled pharmaceuticals, possesses the biologic characteristics that can theoretically allow its prospective validation as a powerful and useful imaging biomarker. One of the advantages of PET is related to the possibility of giving quantitative information on radiopharmaceuticals' biodistribution inside a living organism. Quantitative measurements require a robust standardization to be reproducible. Reproducing a measurement is of paramount importance to allow the use of imaging biomarkers in multicenter trials, when different PET scanners are used in different centers.

STANDARDIZATION PROGRAMS RUNNING IN 2014

There are several studies confirming ^{18}F-fludeoxygluocose (FDG) in different pathologies as a useful PET tracer for the staging of several tumors, but also for the definition of tumor biologic characteristics, for prognosis assessment, and for monitoring patient's response to pharmacologic and radiation therapy. The European Association of Nuclear Medicine[1] (EANM) published procedure guidelines[2] and can be considered one of the standards for the acquisition and reconstruction of PET and PET/computed tomographic (CT) images with

The authors declare no conflict of interest.

Nuclear Medicine Department, Humanitas Clinical and Research Institute, Via A. Manzoni 56, Rozzano, Milan 20089, Italy

* Corresponding author. Humanitas Clinical and Research Institute, Via A. Manzoni 56, Rozzano, Milan 20089, Italy.

E-mail address: arturo.chiti@humanitas.it

PET Clin 9 (2014) 259–266

http://dx.doi.org/10.1016/j.cpet.2014.03.002

FDG. Similar efforts have been concluded or are ongoing worldwide, again to harmonize acquisition, evaluation, and quantification of FDG-PET studies, particularly when the technology must be used in clinical trials.

In Europe, the research branch of EANM, EARL,[3] set up the FDG-PET/CT accreditation program, which was launched in July 2010, to help imaging sites meet the standard requirements indicated in the EANM guideline. The program was immediately endorsed by the European Organisation for Research and Treatment of Cancer[4] Imaging Group, a leading research-oriented organization in Europe. The objective of the EARL accreditation is to provide a minimum standard of PET/CT scanner performance to harmonize the acquisition and interpretation of PET/CT scans. The program requires imaging sites to perform a strict continuing quality control, making it highly eligible as a participant in multicenter studies. Of course, participation in the EARL program ensures that routine patient examinations are of high quality.

In North America, the Society of Nuclear Medicine and Molecular Imaging[5] started the Clinical Trials Network (CTN) to help facilitate the effective use of molecular imaging radiopharmaceuticals in clinical trials. The program is based on a robust scanner validation program and aims at advancing the use of molecular imaging biomarkers in clinical trials, through standardization not only of imaging acquisition and reconstruction but also of chemistry used in the radiopharmaceutical's synthesis. Among the scopes of this effort is the use of imaging biomarkers for drug development, as well as bringing new radiopharmaceuticals to regulatory approval. This program is less strict than EARL in scanner qualification procedures and has a broader scope, including radiopharmaceuticals production and quality control.

Among CTN programs running in 2014, the "Harmonized PET Reconstructions for Cancer Clinical Trials" is a 5-year project, started in September 2012. The program is working to identify and implement harmonized PET reconstruction parameters for all PET/CT scanners to be used in clinical trial scenarios, where quantitative accuracy is critical.

One of the few examples of non-FDG radiopharmaceuticals standardization efforts is the "Gallium-68 Users Group," formed to advance the use of peptide imaging agents in the United States. Members of the Users Group developed harmonized release criteria, an imaging manual, generic data collection forms, and a draft of an informed consent form to aid the participating

centers and the nuclear medicine community at large in establishing investigator-sponsored trials.

The Radiological Society of North America[6] recently founded the Quantitative Imaging Biomarkers Alliance[7] (QIBA), which has the mission to "Improve the value and practicality of quantitative biomarkers by reducing variability across devices, patients and time." This alliance is not focused on PET techniques only, but embraces all imaging techniques, having programs on CT perfusion as well. Within the QIBA framework, a group of experts coming not only from North America but also from all over the world proposed the Uniform Protocols In Clinical Trials document. The goal of this document is: "To facilitate the development and maintenance of widely acceptable, consistent imaging protocols (including imaging quality control procedures) for use in clinical trials across a range of disease states, anatomic sites, and imaging modalities." In particular, the document aims at improving the contribution of imaging data in clinical trials, including improved statistical power while supporting robust case accrual and decreasing time to study initiation/site activation; facilitating image data aggregation across trials; allowing the development, optimization, and validation of imaging biomarkers through the participation of imaging scientists and clinical trialists drawn from the broad range of interested constituencies.

Having sketched the landscape of standardization programs running worldwide, it is clear that, besides the CTN program on ^{68}Ga-DOTA-TOC PET/CT, there is little evidence on the application of standards to non-FDG tracers. Although fluorine-18-labeled radiopharmaceuticals may benefit from the standards that were set up for FDG, radiopharmaceuticals labeled with other positron emitting radionuclides, like carbon-11, gallium-68, nitrogen-13, oxygen-15, copper-64, and zirconium-89, require a specific standard for their reproducibility. It is true for all the requirements that a center needs to participate in a clinical trial, from radiopharmaceutical production to images reporting.

The Japanese Society of Nuclear Medicine[8] is also making an effort to facilitate high-quality research in Japan to acquire data for PET/CT procedure approval, by implementing site audit and qualification programs for in-house production of ^{11}C-methionine (MET) and for imaging with brain tumor phantom (Michio Senda, MD, PhD, Director, Division of Molecular Imaging, Institute of Biomedical Research and Innovation, Kobe, Japan, personal communication, 2012).

This program is aiming for standardization and quality assurance of radiopharmaceuticals produced in hospitals, without any marketing authorization. The main points are guidelines and qualification programs for research using in-house-produced radiopharmaceuticals, such as MET and ^{11}C-Pittsburgh compound B (PiB) and ^{18}F-FDG; training programs; audit and qualification sites; quality control guidelines for PET scanners and imaging procedure; standardization of imaging procedure and scanning protocol; standardization and quality control of PET imaging. It should be emphasized that in Japan FDG is mainly produced in hospitals' radiopharmacies, so it is considered a drug without marketing authorization.

EXAMPLES OF 2 NONSTANDARD PROCEDURES USING CARBON-11 RADIOPHARMACEUTICALS

In this article, some criteria are summarized that aims at optimizing acquisition and interpretation parameters for PET/CT imaging with non-FDG radiopharmaceuticals, after several years of experience in the authors' center.

All the information reported regarding radiopharmaceuticals in this document is related to specific authorization of use, issued by the competent authority in our country to our center and cannot be considered valid for any other center. National and local rules on radiopharmaceuticals preparation and use must be respected by any single center performing PET studies for clinical or research purposes.

There are some aspects that must be considered when doing PET/CT imaging, in general:

- Patient preparation should be as homogeneous as possible, to avoid misleading findings caused by modifications of physiologic radiopharmaceutical biodistribution.
- Radiopharmaceutical administration should be performed according to a strict protocol, which includes timing and instrument cross-calibration.
- Administered activity must be tuned on the clinical question to which the PET/CT study should answer. In Europe, Directive 97/43/EURATOM must be taken into account and recommended national activities for radiopharmaceuticals should not be exceeded for standard procedures.
- There should be particular attention to image quality, calculating radiopharmaceutical activity as a function of patient characteristics, scanner type, scanning mode, and time of acquisition.
- PET and CT parameters for brain and total body acquisition, and reconstruction, must be set according to manufacturer recommendation and national and international guidelines. Those parameters are also set according to patients' characteristics and clinical needs. The justification principle of radiation protection must always be considered, before using any radiation-emitting device or radiopharmaceutical for medical purposes. An example of possible differences between 2 scanners is given in **Table 1**.
- Acquisition protocols should be standardized so that PET/CT images acquired in different centers can be compared and also used in multicenter clinical research protocols.
- Physicians must be aware of the normal tracer distribution and the most important pitfalls that can lead to interpretation errors.
- Reporting should be as homogeneous as possible, stressing the most important clinical findings and giving conclusions able to guide further clinical decisions.
- If previous PET/CT examinations were performed, the images and the reports should be available for comparison.
- In the case of a patient suffering from claustrophobia or not able to maintain the required position for imaging acquisition, technologists must be informed to take necessary actions before the acquisition.
- In case of pregnancy or breast-feeding, specific guidelines must be followed.
- If diagnostic contrast-enhanced CT with intravenous contrast media needs to be performed after the PET/CT examination, a qualified physician must evaluate the indications and contraindications.

Therefore, 2 carbon-11-labeled radiopharmaceuticals are focused on, which are used in the authors' center: ^{11}C-choline (CHO) for prostate cancer and MET for brain tumors.

MET

MET is the most popular amino acid tracer used in PET imaging of brain tumors, because of the low physiologic uptake of MET in brain. Other amino acid PET tracers have entered clinical usage, but MET is the most frequently used, because of its convenient radiochemical production, which allows rapid synthesis with high radiochemical yield without the need for purification steps.[9] Increased uptake of methionine has been shown to correlate with both cellular proliferation[10] and microvessel count[11] in gliomas. After injection, MET uptake in the brain is generally low and, in combination with high tumor uptake, this provides a rationale

Table 1
PET-CT/CT imaging with MET for brain studies and with carbon-11 choline for total body studies (Practical example of different parameters used with 2 different scanners. These examples must be taken in consideration as a starting point given by a particular center, with its own experience.)

Brain Imaging

Scanner A		Scanner B	
CT protocol		**CT protocol**	
Topogram	50 mA 110 kV 256 mm	Topogram	10 mA 120 kV 250 mm
Dose modulation parameters	80 mA 130 kV	Dose modulation parameters	280 mA, maximum value 140 kV
Slice	3 mm	Slice	3.75 mm
Collimation	6 × 2 mm	Collimation	64 × 3.75 mm
Rotation time	1.0 s	Rotation time	1 s
Pitch	1.0	Pitch	0.984:1
Reconstruction for attenuation correction	H10s very smooth 3 mm, FOV 300 mm	Reconstruction for attenuation correction	AC wide view 3.75 mm, FOV 500 mm
Reconstruction for imaging	H31s medium smooth+ 3 mm, FOV 250 mm	Reconstruction for imaging	Standard wide view 0.625 mm, FOV 500 mm
PET protocol		**PET protocol**	
Scan duration bed	10 min	Scan duration bed	10 min
Matrix	256	Matrix	256
Zoom	2	Dfov	30 cm
Reconstruction	Iterations 2; subsets 8	Reconstruction	VUE Point FX, iterations 3, cutoff 4 mm, subset 18, Sharp IRON
Filter	Gaussian	Filter	No filter axis Z
FWHM	4 mm	FWHM	/

Total-Body Imaging

Scanner A		Scanner B	
CT protocol		**CT protocol**	
Topogram	50 mA 110 kV >1000 mm	Topogram	10 mA 120 kV >1000 mm
Dose modulation parameters	95 mA 130 kV	Dose modulation parameters	400 mA, maximum value 140 kV
Slice	3 mm	Slice	3.75 mm
Collimation	6 × 3 mm	Collimation	64 × 3.75 mm
Rotation time	1.0 s	Rotation time	0.5 s
Pitch	1.0	Pitch	0.984
Reconstruction for attenuation correction	B10s very smooth 4 mm, FOV 700 mm	Reconstruction for attenuation correction	AC wide view 3.75 mm, FOV 700 mm
Reconstruction for imaging	B31s medium smooth+ 3 mm	Reconstruction for imaging	Standard wide view 2.5 mm
PET protocol		**PET protocol**	
Scan duration bed	>2.0 min	Scan duration bed	>1.5 min
Matrix	128	Matrix	256
Zoom	1	Dfov	70 cm

(continued on next page)

Table 1 (continued)			
Total-Body Imaging			
Scanner A		**Scanner B**	
Reconstruction	Iterations 2; subset 8	Reconstruction	VUE Point FX, iterations 3, cutoff 5, subset 24, Sharp IRON
Filter	Gaussian	Filter	Standard axis Z
FWHM	4 mm	FWHM	/

Abbreviations: AC, attenuation correction; DFOV, display field of view; FOV, field of view; FWHM, full width half maximum; IRON, general electric proprietary name; VUE Point FX, general electric proprietary name.
Scanner A is from 2006, with no time-of-Flight and a 6-slice CT. Scanner B is from 2012, with time-of-flight and a 64-slice CT.

for the use of MET in the imaging of brain tumors, with an expected high detection rate and good lesion delineation.[12] **Fig. 1** shows an example of the high contrast images that can be obtained with this radiopharmaceutical.

Patient Preparation

- The indication for appropriate use of MET imaging should be evaluated before scheduling the examination.
- On the day of the examination, the patient is asked to fast for at least 4 hours before the radiopharmaceutical administration.
- The physician in charge of the patient may request to withdraw specific drugs during previous clinical evaluations.
- Patient height and body weight and the principal clinical details should be recorded, in particular:
  - Tumor type
  - Known tumor localizations
  - Previous therapies (nature and timing of surgeries, chemotherapy, radiation therapy, or others)
- The radiopharmaceutical is administered as a bolus by intravenous injection followed by flushing with physiologic saline solution. After the administration, the patient needs to wait 10 minutes before scanning.

Administered Activity

Activities of 300 ± 10% MBq are recommended.

Image Interpretation

Normal biodistribution
MET uptake results are low in all cerebral cortex, cerebellum, basal ganglia, and thalamus. Moderate accumulation is observed in pituitary and glandular system (parotid and salivary glands).

Pathologic findings
In the last decade, many studies have evaluated the role of MET PET in primary gliomas

A
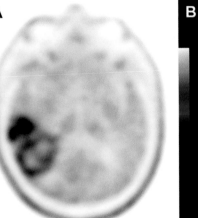

B
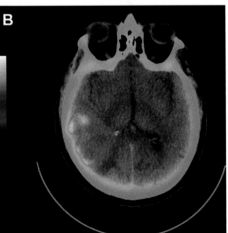

Fig. 1. MET PET/CT highlighting an area of increased uptake in right temporoparietal region, consistent with disease relapse after surgery and radiotherapy. (*A*) PET image. (*B*) PET/CT fused image.

establishing its utility in terms of diagnostic accuracy, prognosis, radiotherapy planning, and biopsy planning. The visual assessment of MET PET images is straightforward and easy. Every area of uptake higher than the background is considered potentially pathologic.

The first quantification method routinely used is the tumor-to-normal background ratio (T/N ratio), comparing the uptake in the tumor to that in the contralateral frontal lobe or the corresponding contralateral hemisphere. Generally, a threshold greater than 1.5 to 1.9 is used for the diagnosis of brain tumor, but large prospective studies are needed to set a fixed T/N cutoff ratio. Uptake may also be defined in terms of the standardized uptake value (SUV). Which SUV should be used (maximum or mean) and if the SUV itself has a real diagnostic value are still a matter of debate.[13] SUV is influenced by scan starting time. MET accumulation in brain tumors reaches a plateau at 5 to 10 minutes after the radiopharmaceutical injection[14,15]; after the plateau phase is reached, the SUV of tumor and normal tissues might be independent of the scan initiation time.[16] Another factor influencing the SUV of MET is the plasma concentrations of N-acetylaspartate (NAA). MET is transported through the NAA transporter from the plasma to the tissues. Therefore, plasma NAA concentrations could affect the uptake of MET in a competitive fashion. However, no previous studies have investigated the effects of plasma NAA concentrations on MET accumulation in the target tissues.[17]

CHO

Prostate cancer is one of the most common malignancies in men and the incidence of prostate cancer increases directly with age. This tumor shows variable biologic behavior, from a clinically silent, indolent intraprostatic tumor to an aggressive malignancy, and causes death in a relatively small proportion of men. Therefore, identifying aggressiveness early in the disease process could be beneficial for therapeutic decision-making.[18,19]

Prostate cancer cells show increased phosphocholine levels and elevated turnover of the cell membrane phospholipid, namely phosphatidylcholine.[20] A high-affinity transporter system imports choline into the cell where it is phosphorylated by choline kinase in the first step of the Kennedy cycle. Key enzymes in choline metabolism, such as choline kinase, are up-regulated in prostate cancers, and this is likely the primary reason prostate cancers concentrate carbon-11 choline.[21]

A major advantage of CHO is its rapid blood clearance (5 min) and rapid uptake within prostate tissue (3–5 min), allowing for early imaging before excretion of the radiotracer into the urine. Thus, the pelvis can be viewed before significant excretory activity becomes a potential confounder. Unfortunately, the 20-minute half-life of carbon-11 restricts the use of CHO to centers with an onsite cyclotron. In contrast, the longer half-life of fluorine-18 (110 min) allows transportation of ^{18}F-fluorocholine to centers without a cyclotron,[22] although ^{18}F-choline has a higher urinary excretion than CHO.[22]

Patient Preparation

- The indication for appropriate use of choline imaging should be evaluated before scheduling the examination.
- On the day of the examination, the patient should be asked to fast at least 4 hours before injection.
- The physician in charge of the patient may request to withdraw specific drugs during previous clinical evaluations.
- Patient height and body weight and the principal clinical details are recorded, in particular:
  ○ Tumor type
  ○ PSA value
  ○ Known tumor localizations
  ○ Previous therapies (kind and time of surgery, chemotherapy, radiation therapy, or monotherapy or others)

The radiopharmaceutical is administered as a bolus by intravenous injection, followed by flushing with physiologic saline solution. After the administration, the patient needs to wait 10 minutes before the scan starts.

Administered Activity

Activities of 350 ± MBq are recommended.

Image Interpretation

Normal biodistribution
Physiologically increased uptake of CHO is noted in salivary glands, liver, kidney parenchyma, and pancreas and faint uptake in spleen, bone marrow, and muscles. Bowel activity is variable. Patients should be well hydrated.

Pathologic findings
The first indication of CHO PET/CT is the local disease evaluation. The high uptake of choline in prostate cancer seems to be caused by active incorporation of choline in tumor cells for production of phosphatidyl choline, a cell membrane constituent, to facilitate rapid cell duplication of tumor cells. Also, normal cells of the prostate actively incorporate choline and produce phosphatidylcholine.[23]

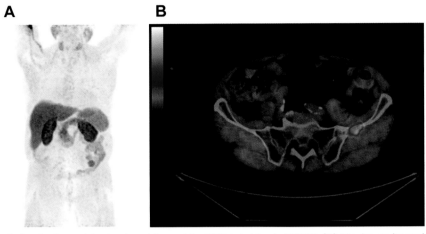

Fig. 2. A bone lesion in the pelvis clearly evidenced by CHO total-body PET/CT. (*A*) Maximum intensity projection image, depicting focal uptake in the left pelvis. (*B*) Axial PET/CT image, localizing the lytic lesion in the left pelvic bone.

Choline uptake is similar in patients with benign prostatic diseases and proven prostate cancer; this is the major limitation for the use of this tracer in identifying the primary tumor, in addition to the limited spatial resolution of PET/CT. Most groups have not found a significant correlation between CHO SUVmax and PSA levels, Gleason score, or disease stage.[24]

SUV is affected by many factors, such as patient size, time between tracer injection, and PET/CT scan. It is possible also to calculate the ratio between SUVmax of the prostate lesion (P) and the pelvis muscles (M), (SUVmax P/M). In a recent study of Chen and colleagues,[25] SUVmax P/M ratio was significantly associated with clinical tumor stage and Gleason score.

Choline PET/CT is a powerful tool for the restaging of biochemically recurrent prostate cancer, particularly for those patients in whom standard imaging (CT, MR imaging, and bone scan) has failed to identify the site of recurrence. This subgroup of patients frequently has one or more lymph node metastases in the pelvis that are normal in size by anatomic imaging, and often there is high tracer uptake in these disease locations.

Choline PET/CT is an optimal imaging modality for the assessment of viable prostate cancer burden in the skeleton (**Fig. 2**); one or more non-sclerotic skeletal metastases are identified, as high focal uptake that can be beyond the field of view of the pelvic MR imaging.[26] It has been clearly demonstrated that choline PET/CT has better sensitivity than bone scan,[27] because choline directly accumulates in the tumor cells in the bone marrow and can detect lesions earlier, whereas bone-seeking radiopharmaceuticals accumulate in the osteoblastic cells as an indirect sign of metastatic disease.

SUMMARY

Standardization of FDG PET-CT is becoming a reality, at least in centers that perform clinical trials. Non-FDG radiopharmaceuticals used with PET/CT are far from standard in clinical trials and in clinical use. This article only gives an example of different protocols and indications related to the availability of different radiopharmaceuticals. This scenario will be probably the reality in the near future in many centers throughout the world. Starting from the FDG experience, it will be easy to implement standards for acquisition and interpretation of PET/CT studies with other radiopharmaceuticals.

REFERENCES

1. Available at: http://www.eanm.org. Accessed January 31, 2014.
2. Boellaard R, O'Doherty MJ, Weber WA, et al. FDG PET and PET/CT: EANM procedure guidelines for tumour PET imaging: version 1.0 EANM guidelines. Eur J Nucl Med Mol Imaging 2010;37:181–200.
3. Available at: http://earl.eanm.org. Accessed January 31, 2014.
4. Available at: http://www.eortc.be. Accessed January 31, 2014.
5. Available at: http://www.snmmi.org. Accessed January 31, 2014.
6. Available at: http://www.rsna.org. Accessed January 31, 2014.
7. Available at: http://qibawiki.rsna.org. Accessed January 31, 2014.

8. Available at: http://www.jsnm.org/english/. Accessed January 31, 2014.

9. Langstrom B, Antoni G, Gullberg P, et al. Synthesis of L- and D-[methyl-11C]methionine. J Nucl Med 1987;28:1037–40.

10. Chung JK, Kim YK, Kim SK, et al. Usefulness of 11C-methionine PET in the evaluation of brain lesions that are hypo- or isometabolic on 18F-FDG PET. Eur J Nucl Med Mol Imaging 2002;29:176–82.

11. Kracht LW, Friese M, Herholz K, et al. Methyl-[11C]-l-methionine uptake as measured by positron emission tomography correlates to microvessel density in patients with glioma. Eur J Nucl Med Mol Imaging 2003;30:868–73.

12. Moulin-Romsee G, D'Hondt E, de Groot T, et al. Non-invasive grading of brain tumours using dynamic amino acid PET imaging: does it work for 11C-methionine? Eur J Nucl Med Mol Imaging 2007;34:2082–7.

13. Glaudemans AW, Enting RH, Heesters MA, et al. Value of 11C-methionine PET in imaging brain tumours and metastases. Eur J Nucl Med Mol Imaging 2013;40:615–35.

14. Lilja A, Bergström K, Hartvig P, et al. Dynamic study of supratentorial gliomas with L-methyl-11C-methionine and positron emission tomography. AJNR Am J Neuroradiol 1985;6:505–14.

15. Kubota K, Matsuzawa T, Ito M, et al. Lung tumor imaging by positron emission tomography using C-11 L-methionine. J Nucl Med 1985;26:37–42.

16. Hatazawa J, Ishiwata K, Itoh M, et al. Quantitative evaluation of L-[methyl-C-11] methionine uptake in tumor using positron emission tomography. J Nucl Med 1989;30:1809–13.

17. Isohashi K, Shimosegawa E, Kato H, et al. Optimization of [11C]methionine PET study: appropriate scan timing and effect of plasma amino acid concentrations on the SUV. EJNMMI Res 2013;3:27.

18. Albersen PC. A challenge to contemporary management of prostate cancer. Nat Clin Pract Urol 2009;6:12–3.

19. Avazpour I, Roslan RE, Bayat P, et al. Segmenting CT images of bronchogenic carcinoma with bone metastases using PET intensity markers approach. Radiol Oncol 2009;43:180–6.

20. Ackerstaff E, Glunde K, Bhujwalla ZM. Choline phospholipid metabolism: a target in cancer cells? J Cell Biochem 2003;90:525–33.

21. Farsad M, Schiavina R, Castelluci P, et al. Detection and localization of prostate cancer: correlation of (11)C-choline PET/CT with histopathologic step-section analysis. J Nucl Med 2005;46:1642–9.

22. Hara T, Kosaka N, Kishi H. PET imaging of prostate cancer using carbon-11-choline. J Nucl Med 1998;39:990–5.

23. Pulido JA, del Hoyo N, Pérez-Albarsanz MA. Composition and fatty acid content of rat ventral prostate phospholipids. Biochim Biophys Acta 1986;879:51–5.

24. Giovacchini G, Picchio M, Coradeschi E, et al. [11C]Choline uptake with PET/CT for the initial diagnosis of prostate cancer: relation to PSA levels, tumour stage and anti-androgenic therapy. Eur J Nucl Med Mol Imaging 2008;35:1065–73.

25. Chen J, Zhao Y, Li X, et al. Imaging primary prostate cancer with 11C-Choline PET/CT: relation to tumour stage, Gleason score and biomarkers of biologic aggressiveness. Radiol Oncol 2012;46(3):179–88.

26. Murphy RC, Kawashima A, Peller PJ. The utility of 11C-choline PET/CT for imaging prostate cancer: a pictorial guide. AJR Am J Roentgenol 2011;196:1390–8.

27. Fuccio C, Castellucci P, Schiavina R, et al. Role of (11)C-choline PET/CT in the re-staging of prostate cancer patients with biochemical relapse and negative results at bone scintigraphy. Eur J Radiol 2012;81:893–6.

Brain: Positron Emission Tomography Tracers Beyond [18F] Fluorodeoxyglucose

Tarun Singhal, MD[a], Abass Alavi, MD[b], Chun K. Kim, MD[a],*

KEYWORDS

- Positron emission tomography • Brain • Central nervous system • Positron • Dementia
- Parkinson disease • Epilepsy • Neuroinflammation

KEY POINTS

- Positron emission tomography (PET) has led to significant insights into nervous system biology, physiology, and pathophysiology in health and disease.
- Several PET radiopharmaceuticals beyond fluorodeoxyglucose (FDG) have been used to study the physiology and pathophysiology in neurosciences.
- Future studies on the use of advanced PET imaging in delineating neural pathophysiology, drug development, and altering patient management and outcomes across the disciplines of neurosciences are needed.

INTRODUCTION

Positron emission tomography (PET) is a molecular imaging technique used for generating maps of functional and biochemical activity in target tissues in vivo.[1] PET has led to significant insights into nervous system biology, physiology, and pathophysiology in health and disease. Several of these insights and applications have a direct usefulness for the neurologist.[2] Although fluorine 18 [18F]fluorodeoxyglucose (FDG) has remained a workhorse of clinical PET imaging, many other radiolabeled biomolecules have been studied using PET.[3] In this article, brain PET ligands beyond FDG, across the spectrum of neurologic subspecialties, including dementias, movement disorders, epilepsy, brain tumors, and neuroinflammation, are reviewed. Of the numerous available PET radiopharmaceuticals, a few have been selected that have been extensively studied in common neurologic disorders.

DEMENTIA

There is widespread deposition of amyloid in the cerebral cortex in Alzheimer disease (AD). Carbon 11 (^{11}C) Pittsburgh compound B (PiB) is a radiolabeled analogue of thioflavin dye, which has been established as a valid biomarker for amyloid deposition in the human brain.[4] Given the short half-life of ^{11}C, limiting its availability, several ^{18}F-labeled amyloid-binding PET radiopharmaceuticals have been developed, including ^{18}F-florbetapir, ^{18}F-flutemetamol and ^{18}F-florbetaben, which have recently been approved by the US Food and Drug Administration (FDA) for clinical use.[5–7] However, no single diagnostic test or imaging is considered sufficient. Amyloid imaging and cerebrospinal fluid CSF Aβ levels are considered markers of the neuropathologic process, whereas FDG-PET is considered a marker for neuronal damage, and their combined interpretation may aid a diagnosis of AD in the right clinical context.[8]

Author Disclosures: None.
[a] Division of Nuclear Medicine and Molecular Imaging, Department of Radiology, Brigham and Women's Hospital, Harvard Medical School, 75 Francis Street, Boston, MA 02115, USA; [b] Division of Nuclear Medicine, Department of Radiology, University of Pennsylvania School of Medicine, Hospital of the University of Pennsylvania, Philadelphia, Pennsylvania
* Corresponding author. Division of Nuclear Medicine and Molecular Imaging, Department of Radiology, Brigham and Women's Hospital, Harvard Medical School, 75 Francis Street, ASB1 L1-037, Boston, MA 02115.
E-mail address: ckkim@bwh.harvard.edu

PET Clin 9 (2014) 267–276
http://dx.doi.org/10.1016/j.cpet.2014.03.009
1556-8598/14/$ – see front matter © 2014 Elsevier Inc. All rights reserved.

There has been a controversy regarding the overall and relative usefulness of these PET agents with respect to FDG-PET for diagnosing AD.[9–11]

[18]F-Florbetapir is a fluorine-labeled stilbene derivative. The recommended dose for ^{18}F-florbetapir is 370 MBq (10 mCi). For routine clinical use, the scan is obtained as a 10-minute acquisition, starting 40 to 50 minutes after intravenous injection (**Table 1**). The effective radiation dose after a 10-mCi injection in an adult is 7.0 mSv.[12] An excellent correlation between ^{18}F-florbetapir and ^{11}C-PiB uptake has been shown.[13]

Normal amyloid scans show a clear gray-white matter contrast, with more radioactivity concentration in white matter. In patients with AD, uptake is increased in the orbitofrontal cortex, anterior cingulate, precuneus, posterior cingulate, and lateral temporal cortex, consistent with autopsy findings in direct comparison studies (**Fig. 1**).[2,14] According to some recommendations, the ^{18}F-florbetapir scan is considered positive if either (1) 2 or more brain areas (each larger than a single cortical gyrus) show reduced or absent gray-white matter contrast, or (2) there are 1 or more areas in which gray matter uptake is intense and clearly exceeds the uptake in adjacent white matter. A potential pitfall of scan interpretation using these criteria is in cases with brain atrophy, in which the gray-white matter contrast may be lost because of atrophy rather than abnormal accumulation in the gray matter. Alternatively, the ratio of radiotracer concentration in the region of disease to either the whole brain or to pons has been proposed as a semiquantitative index of ^{18}F-florbetapir uptake.[15]

On correlation with disease, a negative amyloid scan corresponded to a neuropathologic amyloid deposition rating (Consortium to Establish a Registry for Alzheimer's Disease) of none to sparse, whereas a positive amyloid scan corresponded to a rating of moderate to frequent amyloid plaque deposition in the cortex.

Amyloid imaging can be useful in differentiating AD from frontotemporal dementia. Patients with frontotemporal dementia do not show significant amyloid deposition. However, abnormal amyloid deposition may be seen in 50% to 70% of patients with dementia with Lewy bodies (DLB) (**Table 2**).[16] Negative ^{18}F-florbetapir PET scans have been reported for some clinically diagnosed patients with AD, consistent with literature reports that 10% to 20% of clinically diagnosed patients with AD do not have amyloid disease at autopsy.[17]

False-positive results may be obtained in apparently healthy persons and are found in 12% of those in their 60s, 30% of those in their 70s, and approximately 50% of those older than 80 years.[16] Carriers of the ApoE-4 allele, constituting 27% of the general population, have almost 3 times the risk of a positive ^{11}C-PiB scan, even if cognitively normal, and a similar increase in the risk of developing AD. Overall accuracy of amyloid imaging for AD is estimated to be more than 90% for patients younger than 70 years, about 85% for patients in their 70s, and 75% to 80% for those older than 80 years.[16]

Amyloid imaging also has a role in evaluation of patients with mild cognitive impairment (MCI). Patients with MCI have a 70% chance of progression to AD over a 3-year period if the amyloid scan is read as positive, as opposed to only a 10% chance if the scan is deemed to be negative. Similarly, there is a high likelihood of AD being a cause of

---

Table 1
Imaging protocols

[18]F-Florbetapir	10-min acquisition starting 40–50 min after intravenous injection of 10 mCi
[11]C- or ^{18}F-Flumazenil	Dynamic list mode acquisition for 60–90 min after injection of 10 mCi
[11]C-Methionine or ^{18}F-fluoroethyltyrosine	Dynamic acquisition or 10-min acquisition performed 20 min after injection of 10 mCi
[18]F-Fluorothymidine	Dynamic acquisition obtained for 60–90 min after injection of radiopharmaceutical or static imaging obtained for 10 min 60 min after injection of 5–10 mCi
[18]F-Fluorodopa	Ki values obtained from dynamic imaging performed over 90 min. Static imaging performed 60–70 min after injection for striatal imaging in movement disorders but earlier (approximately 20 min) for brain tumor evaluation
[18]F-Fluoropropyl-(+)-dihydrotetrabenazine	10-min acquisition 90 min after intravenous injection of 10 mCi or dynamic acquisition
[11]C-PK11195	Dynamic acquisition over approximately 60 min

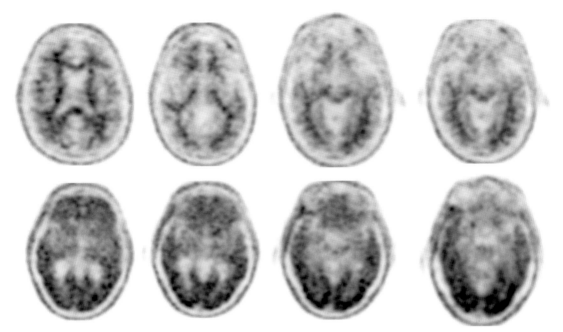

Fig. 1. (*Top row*) Normal ^{18}F-florbetapir amyloid scan showing clear gray-white matter contrast with higher uptake in white matter. (*Bottom row*) Positive ^{18}F-florbetapir amyloid scan with extensive loss of gray-white matter contrast.

Table 2 Pearls, pitfalls, variants	
Amyloid agents	50%–70% of patients with DLB may have positive scans 10%–20% of patients with AD may have negative scans False-positive results in 12%, 30%, and 50% of normal adults in 60s, 70s, 80s age group, respectively
^{11}C- or ^{18}F-Flumazenil	Patients with coma and vegetative state, motor neuron disease, cerebral ischemia may have decreased flumazenil binding Increased levels of flumazenil may be seen in white matter, reflecting microdysgenesis
^{11}C-Methionine or ^{18}F-fluoroethyltyrosine	False-positive results may be seen in benign conditions such as demyelination, leukoencephalitis, or abscess Major clinical usefulness in determination of tumor extent, treatment, and biopsy planning and detection of low-grade gliomas
^{18}F-Fluorothymidine	Predominantly taken up in tumor regions with a disrupted blood-brain barrier Lower sensitivity than methionine PET for low-grade gliomas
^{18}F-Fluorodopa	Underestimation of degree of neuronal degeneration in early PD caused by upregulation of AADC enzyme
^{18}F-FP-(+)-dihydrotetrabenazine	Asymmetric decline in binding in PD, most severe contralateral to symptomatic side Decreased striatal uptake also seen in DLB
^{11}C-PK11195	Increased binding seen in multiple sclerosis, AD, PD, DLB, neuropsychiatric illnesses Nonspecific binding and poor signal/contrast ratio complicates quantification

Abbreviations: AD, Alzheimer disease; DLB, dementia with Lewy bodies; FP, fluoropropyl; PD, Parkinson disease.

MCI when both an amyloid and a neurodegenerative biomarker for AD (such as hypometabolism on FDG-PET or increased phospho-tau levels in CSF) are positive, intermediate likelihood if just 1 biomarker is tested and that is positive, or MCI is unlikely to be caused by AD if both amyloid and neurodegenerative biomarkers are negative.[18] Although there is a positive correlation between the degree of amyloid uptake and cognitive decline in MCI, it is not the case in patients with AD.[16]

EPILEPSY

Several radiopharmaceuticals other than FDG have been studied in epilepsy. Most data are available for ^{11}C-flumazenil PET and ^{11}C-α-methyl tryptophan PET.[2] Recently, results with ^{18}F-flumazenil have also been reported.[19]

Flumazenil is a specific benzodiazepine antagonist, which is reversibly bound at the benzodiazepine binding sites of γ-aminobutyric acid (GABA)-A receptors containing 4 of the 6 possible α subunits: α_1, α_2, α_3, and α_5. These subunits are the most prevalent subunits of the GABA-A receptors, and most neurons express GABA-A receptors, so radiolabeled flumazenil can be considered a neuronal marker as well.[20,21] The bulk of normal binding of radiolabeled flumazenil is principally in the neocortex, with lower binding in the hippocampus, cerebellum, and subcortical structures, including the thalamus and basal ganglia.[20,22]

Fully quantitative estimates of volume of distribution using arterial input function or image-derived input function (with kinetic modeling using a reference tissue model) have been compared with semiquantitative indices obtained from integrating data over different time points during dynamic acquisitions of about 90 minutes, after intravenous injection of approximately 370 MBq (10 mCi) of ^{11}C-flumazenil (see **Table 1**).[23] The other indices often reported in various studies include receptor density (B_{max}) and receptor affinity (Kd). Recently, results have been reported for ^{18}F-flumazenil in patients with refractory epilepsy without the use of arterial input function.[19] Images are interpreted from asymmetry or compared with a reference normal population of healthy controls. In focal epilepsies, an average reduction of 30% has been reported in the GABA-A receptor density in the epileptogenic focus using ^{11}C-flumazenil.[20] This finding is independent of loss of neuronal tissue and also detected when magnetic resonance (MR) imaging volumes are normal. Correction for partial volume effects is considered mandatory when structural changes are present in the afflicted population, for example, in hippocampal sclerosis or mesial temporal sclerosis.

Neuropathologic studies have shown a reduction in number of GABA-A receptors over and above neuronal loss in the CA1 region of hippocampus, which is the most severely affected in patients with classic hippocampal sclerosis (along with the CA4 region, and as opposed to the CA2 region, which is also known as the resistant sector). However, in the other regions, the reduction was congruent to the neuronal loss.[20,24]

Increases of ^{11}C-flumazenil binding may be seen in the white matter that correlates with the number of heterotopic neurons, reflecting microdysgenesis. Similar findings may be seen in patients with malformations of cortical development (see **Table 2**). These patients may have normal MR imaging evaluations and may suffer from potential treatment failure after surgical resection if only the cortical lesion detected on MR imaging (eg, hippocampal sclerosis) is resected. Similarly, occult neuronal migration disorders not identified on MR imaging, may play a key role in the pathophysiology of cryptogenic focal epilepsies. PET imaging with radiolabeled flumazenil is a potential powerful tool for identifying these patients. These findings may be missed if only semiquantitative data or asymmetry indices are used, and hence, kinetic modeling may be required.[20]

Epileptogenic foci identified by flumazenil-PET tend to be smaller than the areas of hypometabolism on FDG-PET (**Fig. 2**).[19,20,25] The degree of decreased ^{11}C-flumazenil binding has been shown to correlate with seizure frequency, but this finding is controversial.[20,26] False lateralization may be seen in contralateral temporal lobe after a seizure, reflecting rapid neuronal plasticity with respect to GABA-A receptors after a seizure.[27]

Reduced flumazenil binding has been reported in areas of disease in patients with coma and vegetative state, motor neuron disease, and cerebral ischemia (see **Table 2**).[28–30] It is, hence, important to obtain a complete neurologic history before interpretation of scans performed for evaluation of epilepsy.

[11]C-α-Methyl tryptophan is another PET radiopharmaceutical used for evaluation of patients with epilepsy. This tracer studies cellular incorporation of the amino acids. Unlike FDG or flumazenil, increased uptake of ^{11}C-α-methyl tryptophan is seen in epileptic foci, particularly in patients with tuberous sclerosis and cortical developmental malformations.[31,32]

MOVEMENT DISORDERS

Characteristic patterns of nigrostriatal projection abnormalities have been identified in movement disorders. Presynaptic dopaminergic imaging

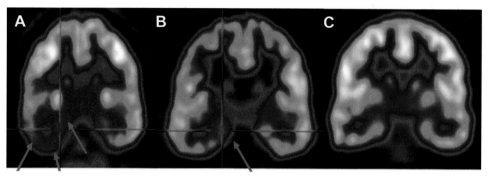

Fig. 2. (*A*) FDG-PET scan showing extensive area of hypometabolism in right temporal lobe (*arrows*). (*B*) ^{18}F-Flumazenil PET image shows more restricted localization to mesial temporal region in same patient (*arrow*). (*C*) Symmetric ^{18}F-flumazenil distribution in control individual. (*From* Vivash L, Gregoire MC, Lau EW, et al. 18F-Flumazenil: a g-aminobutyric acid A–specific PET radiotracer for the localization of drug-resistant temporal lobe epilepsy. J Nucl Med 2013;54:1273; with permission.)

can be useful; (1) in distinguishing psychogenic movement disorders from early idiopathic Parkinson disease and (2) for confirming the diagnosis of Parkinson disease in a patient with atypical clinical features such as an early age of onset or to enable distinction from essential tremors.[33,34] The integrity of nigrostriatal projections has been extensively studied with ^{18}F-fluorodopa (FDOPA) PET, which is a marker for presynaptic dopaminergic function. FDOPA uptake depends on its transport across the blood-brain barrier, uptake into dopaminergic neurons, decarboxylation by amino acid decarboxylase enzyme to form ^{18}F-dopamine, vesicular storage of ^{18}F-dopamine, and degradation of ^{18}F-dopamine by monoamine oxidase-B and catechol-o-methyl transferase enzymes. The striatal uptake of FDOPA increases with time, and static imaging is generally performed 60 to 70 minutes after injection. Ki values may be obtained from dynamic imaging (see **Table 1**).[33,35]

There is decreased FDOPA uptake in idiopathic Parkinson disease, which is most prominent in posterior putamen followed by anterior putamen and with relative sparing of the caudate and ventral striatum. The degree of decreased FDOPA uptake correlates with severity of symptoms, particularly rigidity and bradykinesia. However, in early Parkinson disease, FDOPA may underestimate the degree of neuronal degeneration because of compensatory upregulation of amino acid decarboxylase enzyme (see **Table 2**).[36] On the other hand, FDOPA Ki may be increased in globus pallidus at the onset of Parkinson disease, which subsequently decreases as disease progresses. Image analysis using statistical parametric mapping showed areas of increased FDOPA uptake in the dorsolateral prefrontal cortex, anterior cingulate and globus pallidus interna,

which may reflect compensatory changes, seen during early phases of disease.[33]

Vesicular monoamine transporter 2 (VMAT2), a protein responsible for pumping monoamine neurotransmitters from the cytosol into synaptic vesicles, can be imaged with PET using ^{11}C-fluoropropyl (FP) and ^{18}F-FP (+)dihydrotetrabenazine (DTBZ). Dynamic image acquisition protocols have been described for ^{11}C-DTBZ imaging. However, ^{18}F-FP-DTBZ may be obtained as a 10-minute acquisition 90 minutes after injection of 10 mCi of the radiopharmaceutical. Occipital lobe has been used as a reference region in patients with Parkinson disease. The highest binding of DTBZ in normal individuals is seen in putamen, caudate, nucleus accumbens, hypothalamus, substantia nigra, raphe nuclei, locus coeruleus, brain stem, and amygdala, in decreasing order of relative uptake.[37] DTBZ has been shown to be a marker of nigrostriatal terminal density and shows decreased binding in caudate nucleus and anterior and posterior putamen in Parkinson disease and DLB compared with the healthy population and patients with AD.[38] There is significant asymmetry of binding in patients with Parkinson disease, with the most severe reduction seen in the striatum contralateral to the clinically affected side (**Fig. 3**).[38] Analysis of neocortical blood-to-brain ligand transport (K1) estimates obtained from dynamic imaging, combined with estimates of striatal distribution volume using ^{11}C-DTBZ was able to segregate patients with AD, Parkinson disease, and DLB with 90% accuracy in 1 study.[39] A similar approach may be attempted with ^{18}F-FP-DTBZ.

A presynaptic single-photon emission computed tomography (SPECT) agent for dopamine transporter ([I-123] ioflupane) has been recently approved by the FDA for clinical use to distinguish neurodegenerative parkinsonian syndromes from

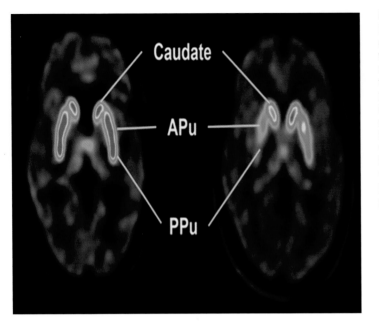

Fig. 3. Representative ^{18}F-DTBZ PET images in a healthy individual (*left*) and patient with PD (*right*). In patient with PD, uptake of ^{18}F-DTBZ was markedly decreased in bilateral striatum, with worst effects in posterior putamen (PPu) contralateral to the symptomatic side as compared to the anterior putamen (APu). (*From* Lin SC, Lin KJ, Hsiao IT, et al. In vivo detection of monoaminergic degeneration in early Parkinson disease by 18F-9-fluoropropyl-(1)-dihydrotetrabenzazine PET. J Nucl Med 2014;55:75; with permission.)

nonneurodegenerative parkinsonism (ie, drug-induced parkinsonism and psychogenic parkinsonism) and essential tremor, based on preserved uptake of the tracer in the latter. Given technical advantages of PET over SPECT, dopamine transporter and VMAT2 PET ligands are expected to become the preferred agents once approved for routine clinical use. The expression of dopamine transporter may be altered by dopaminergic or dopaminomimetic drugs and may not accurately reflect density of dopaminergic terminals in patients with Parkinson disease.[40]

Radiolabeled ligands for dopamine receptors (eg, ^{11}C-raclopride) have been studied for postsynaptic changes in basal ganglia. Although the uptake for these agents is preserved or increased in early Parkinson disease, it is decreased in patients with atypical parkinsonism (multiple system atrophy or progressive supranuclear palsy).[41]

BRAIN TUMORS

Evaluation of brain tumors with FDG-PET is limited by the high background physiologic uptake of FDG. On the other hand, radiolabeled amino acids (eg, ^{11}C-methionine, ^{18}F-fluoroethyltyrosine [FET]) have high uptake in tumors but not in brain parenchyma, thereby providing a good lesion-to-background contrast, which enables a high sensitivity for detecting low-grade gliomas (**Fig. 4**).[42] The increased amino acid uptake has been shown to be a reflection of an upregulation of L-type amino acid transporter 1 (LAT1) and proliferation of the tumor microvasculature. LAT1 is an

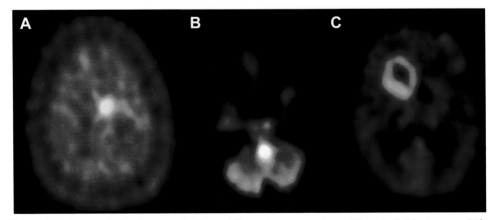

Fig. 4. ^{11}C-Methionine uptake in a low-grade glioma (*A*), grade III astrocytoma (*B*), and glioblastoma multiforme (*C*).

Na-independent amino acid transport system, and a major route for passage of large neutral amino acids through the plasma membrane.[43,44] In high-grade gliomas, tracer leakage from a disrupted blood-brain barrier contributes significantly to the amino acid uptake.[45] However, in low-grade gliomas (noncontrast enhancing), there is amino acid uptake without significant blood-brain barrier breakdown, corresponding to an upregulation of LAT1. On the other hand, FDG-PET has prognostic value above and beyond histopathologic examination across tumor grades, and delayed imaging protocols increase the sensitivity of FDG-PET.[46,47]

In preparation for the radiolabeled amino acid PET scan, patients are advised to take a low-protein diet 4 hours before the injection, although this requirement is controversial (**Table 3**). Imaging may be performed as a dynamic acquisition or static acquisition 20 minutes after injection of 370 to 740 MBq (10–20 mCi) of ^{11}C-methionine or ^{18}F-FET (see **Table 1**).[48]

Although ^{11}C-methionine PET has been shown to have high sensitivity for gliomas, including low-grade gliomas, false-positive results may be seen in benign conditions, such as demyelination, leukoencephalitis, or abscess. Oligodendrogliomas have higher methionine uptake compared with diffuse astrocytomas of similar grade.[42] Using tumor to contralateral normal (T/N) cortex ratio of 1.47 as cutoff, a sensitivity of 76% to 95% and specificity of approximately 87% have been reported for gliomas.[45,49]

A multimodality approach has been suggested for tumor grading and prognostication, using contrast-enhanced MR imaging, ^{11}C-methionine-PET and FDG-PET, in which higher methionine uptake predicted poorer outcome better in low-grade and non–contrast-enhancing gliomas, whereas higher FDG uptake was a better predictor of poorer outcome in high-grade and contrast-enhancing gliomas.[50]

The improved tumor/background ratio with ^{11}C-methionine imaging enables better delineation of tumor margin. The methionine uptake may extend up to more than 30 mm beyond the contrast-enhanced area on the T1-weighted MR imaging in patients with glioblastoma multiforme. In terms of biopsy planning, combined use of MR imaging and FET PET improves the sensitivity to 93% and specificity to 94%, as opposed to 96% sensitivity and only 53% specificity with MR imaging alone. Several studies have shown the usefulness of amino acid imaging in surgical resection and radiation treatment planning. Amino acid PET may also be used for assessing response to treatment and a 15% change (increase or decrease) in T/N ratios is considered significant.[42]

For detection of recurrent tumors using ^{11}C-methionine PET, a recent meta-analysis[51] reported a summary sensitivity of 70% and specificity of 93% for high-grade gliomas. Similar to radiolabeled methionine, FDOPA is an amino acid tracer and accumulates in brain tumors by similar transporter-mediated mechanisms, so the imaging may be performed at an earlier time point after injection (eg, 20 minutes) than is recommended for striatal imaging (eg, 60–70 minutes), as described earlier.[35]

^{18}F-Fluoro-*L*-thymidine (FLT) has been studied as a marker of DNA synthesis in brain tumors. FLT is taken up predominantly in tumor regions with a disrupted blood-brain barrier. For low-grade gliomas, sensitivity of FLT imaging for tumor detection is lower than that of methionine PET (78.3% vs 91.3%) (see **Table 2**). A combination of FLT-PET, methionine PET, and gadolinium-enhanced MR imaging may provide complementary information on the true extent of the tumor.[52]

NEUROINFLAMMATION

Microglia are the resident macrophages of the central nervous system, comprising up to 20% of the nonneuronal cell population of the brain.[53] Microglial activation is known to play a major role in appearance and progression of several

Table 3	
What the referring physician needs to know	
Amyloid agents	No fasting required
^{11}C-Flumazenil	Preferably seizure free for 24 h[a]
^{11}C-Methionine or ^{18}F-fluoroethyltyrosine	Low-protein diet at approximately 4 h before scan[a]
^{18}F-Fluorothymidine	No fasting required
^{18}F-Fluorodopa	Preferably off dopaminergic or dopaminomimetic drugs for minimum 12 h before scan[a]

[a] These recommendations are not standardized but reflect some of the reported practices.

neurologic and psychiatric disorders. Translocator protein (TSPO) is an 18-kDa outer mitochondrial membrane protein, which is upregulated during microglial activation and is also overexpressed in activated macrophages and astrocytes.[54] Several PET ligands have been developed to target TSPO. ^{11}C-PK11195 is the classic agent for TSPO imaging and has been most widely studied, but a high level of nonspecific binding and poor signal-to-noise complicates its quantification. ^{11}C-PBR-28 and ^{18}F-GE-180 are some of the newer neuroinflammation PET imaging markers.[55,56] Interindividual variability complicates interpretation of ^{11}C-PBR28, and genetic polymorphisms accounting for interindividual differences have been described.[57]

Microglial activation has been reported in patients with stroke at the site of primary insult as well as remotely along the white matter tracts.[58] ^{11}C-PK11195 binding in black holes of multiple sclerosis has been found to be a predictor of progressive disability.[59] In patients with AD, there was increased binding of ^{11}C-PBR28 in temporal and parietal cortical brain regions and the degree of binding inversely correlated with performance on cognitive scales and gray matter volumes.[60] This relationship was not seen in patients with MCI, implicating the role of neuroinflammation in the evolution of MCI to AD. In DLB, microglial activation is seen in substantia nigra, putamen, and several association cortical areas using ^{11}C-PK11195, whereas patients with Parkinson disease showed microglial activation only in the substantia nigra and putamen.[61] Higher binding of ^{11}C-PK11195 was reported in the hippocampus of schizophrenic patients, suggesting a role of focal neuroinflammation in its pathophysiology (see **Table 2**).[62] More studies are needed to study the relative merits and demerits of different radiopharmaceuticals for studying neuroinflammation and their potential diagnostic and therapeutic implications.

SUMMARY

Several PET radiopharmaceuticals beyond FDG have been used to study the physiology and pathophysiology in neurosciences. This article provides a broad overview of some of the commonly studied radiopharmaceuticals for PET imaging in selected neurologic conditions, particularly attempting to study their clinical relevance. Future studies on the use of advanced PET imaging in delineating neural pathophysiology, drug development, and altering patient management and outcomes across the disciplines of neurosciences are needed.

REFERENCES

1. Phelps ME. Positron emission tomography provides molecular imaging of biological processes. Proc Natl Acad Sci U S A 2000;97(16):9226–33.
2. Singhal T. Positron emission tomography applications in clinical neurology. Semin Neurol 2012; 32(4):421–31.
3. Jones T, Rabiner EA, PET Research Advisory Company. The development, past achievements, and future directions of brain PET. J Cereb Blood Flow Metab 2012;32(7):1426–54.
4. Klunk WE, Engler H, Nordberg A, et al. Imaging brain amyloid in Alzheimer's disease with Pittsburgh Compound-B. Ann Neurol 2004;55(3): 306–19.
5. Yang L, Rieves D, Ganley C. Brain amyloid imaging–FDA approval of florbetapir F18 injection. N Engl J Med 2012;367(10):885–7.
6. GE beta-amyloid agent approved. J Nucl Med 2013;54(12):10N.
7. Available at: http://www.wmis.org/fda-approves-piramal-imagings-neuraceqtm-florbetaben-f18-injection-for-pet-imaging-of-beta-amyloid-neuritic-plaques-in-the-brain/. Accessed 27 April, 2014.
8. McKhann GM, Knopman DS, Chertkow H, et al. The diagnosis of dementia due to Alzheimer's disease: recommendations from the National Institute on Aging-Alzheimer's Association workgroups on diagnostic guidelines for Alzheimer's disease. Alzheimers Dement 2011;7(3):263–9.
9. Kepe V, Moghbel MC, Långström B, et al. Amyloid-β positron emission tomography imaging probes: a critical review. J Alzheimers Dis 2013;36(4): 613–31.
10. Moghbel MC, Saboury B, Basu S, et al. Amyloid-β imaging with PET in Alzheimer's disease: is it feasible with current radiotracers and technologies? Eur J Nucl Med Mol Imaging 2012;39(2): 202–8.
11. Villemagne VL, Klunk WE, Mathis CA, et al. Aβ Imaging: feasible, pertinent, and vital to progress in Alzheimer's disease. Eur J Nucl Med Mol Imaging 2012;39(2):209–19.
12. Joshi AD, Pontecorvo MJ, Adler L, et al. Radiation dosimetry of florbetapir F 18. EJNMMI Res 2014; 4(1):4. http://dx.doi.org/10.1186/2191-219X-4-4.
13. Wolk DA, Zhang Z, Boudhar S, et al. Amyloid imaging in Alzheimer's disease: comparison of florbetapir and Pittsburgh compound-B positron emission tomography. J Neurol Neurosurg Psychiatry 2012; 83(9):923–6.
14. Choi SR, Schneider JA, Bennett DA, et al. Correlation of amyloid PET ligand florbetapir F 18 binding with abeta aggregation and neuritic plaque deposition in postmortem brain tissue. Alzheimer Dis Assoc Disord 2012;26(1):8–16.

15. Clark CM, Pontecorvo MJ, Beach TG, et al. Cerebral PET with florbetapir compared with neuropathology at autopsy for detection of neuritic amyloid-beta plaques: a prospective cohort study. Lancet Neurol 2012;11(8):669–78.

16. Rowe CC, Villemagne VL. Brain amyloid imaging. J Nucl Med 2011;52(11):1733–40.

17. Lim A, Tsuang D, Kukull W, et al. Clinico-neuropathological correlation of Alzheimer's disease in a community-based case series. J Am Geriatr Soc 1999;47(5):564–9.

18. Albert MS, DeKosky ST, Dickson D, et al. The diagnosis of mild cognitive impairment due to Alzheimer's disease: recommendations from the National Institute on Aging-Alzheimer's Association Workgroups on Diagnostic Guidelines for Alzheimer's Disease. Alzheimers Dement 2011;7(3): 270–9.

19. Vivash L, Gregoire MC, Lau EW, et al. 18F-flumazenil: a gamma-aminobutyric acid A-specific PET radiotracer for the localization of drug-resistant temporal lobe epilepsy. J Nucl Med 2013;54(8): 1270–7.

20. Hammers A. Flumazenil positron emission tomography and other ligands for functional imaging. Neuroimaging Clin N Am 2004;14(3):537–51.

21. Olsen RW, McCabe RT, Wamsley JK. GABAA receptor subtypes: autoradiographic comparison of GABA, benzodiazepine, and convulsant binding sites in the rat central nervous system. J Chem Neuroanat 1990;3(1):59–76.

22. Holthoff VA, Koeppe RA, Frey KA, et al. Differentiation of radioligand delivery and binding in the brain: validation of a two-compartment model for [11C]flumazenil. J Cereb Blood Flow Metab 1991; 11(5):745–52.

23. Hammers A, Panagoda P, Heckemann RA, et al. 11C]flumazenil PET in temporal lobe epilepsy: do we need an arterial input function or kinetic modeling? J Cereb Blood Flow Metab 2008;28(1): 207–16.

24. Koepp MJ, Hand KS, Labbe C, et al. In vivo [11C] flumazenil-PET correlates with ex vivo [3H]flumazenil autoradiography in hippocampal sclerosis. Ann Neurol 1998;43(5):618–26.

25. Muzik O, da Silva EA, Juhasz C, et al. Intracranial EEG versus flumazenil and glucose PET in children with extratemporal lobe epilepsy. Neurology 2000; 54(1):171–9.

26. Savic I, Svanborg E, Thorell JO. Cortical benzodiazepine receptor changes are related to frequency of partial seizures: a positron emission tomography study. Epilepsia 1996;37(3):236–44.

27. Ryvlin P, Bouvard S, Le Bars D, et al. Transient and falsely lateralizing flumazenil-PET asymmetries in temporal lobe epilepsy. Neurology 1999;53(8): 1882–5.

28. Heiss WD. PET in coma and in vegetative state. Eur J Neurol 2012;19(2):207–11.

29. Heiss WD. The ischemic penumbra: how does tissue injury evolve? Ann N Y Acad Sci 2012;1268: 26–34.

30. Turner MR, Leigh PN. Positron emission tomography (PET)–its potential to provide surrogate markers in ALS. Amyotroph Lateral Scler Other Motor Neuron Disord 2000;1(Suppl 2):S17–22.

31. Kagawa K, Chugani DC, Asano E, et al. Epilepsy surgery outcome in children with tuberous sclerosis complex evaluated with alpha-[11C]methyl-L-tryptophan positron emission tomography (PET). J Child Neurol 2005;20(5):429–38.

32. Rubi S, Costes N, Heckemann RA, et al. Positron emission tomography with alpha-[11C]methyl-L-tryptophan in tuberous sclerosis complex-related epilepsy. Epilepsia 2013;54(12):2143–50.

33. Brooks DJ, Pavese N. Imaging biomarkers in Parkinson's disease. Prog Neurobiol 2011;95(4): 614–28.

34. Stoessl AJ, Martin WW, McKeown MJ, et al. Advances in imaging in Parkinson's disease. Lancet Neurol 2011;10(11):987–1001.

35. Becherer A, Karanikas G, Szabo M, et al. Brain tumour imaging with PET: a comparison between [18F]fluorodopa and [11C]methionine. Eur J Nucl Med Mol Imaging 2003;30(11):1561–7.

36. Ishikawa T, Dhawan V, Chaly T, et al. Clinical significance of striatal DOPA decarboxylase activity in Parkinson's disease. J Nucl Med 1996;37(2): 216–22.

37. Lin KJ, Weng YH, Hsieh CJ, et al. Brain imaging of vesicular monoamine transporter type 2 in healthy aging subjects by 18F-FP-(+)-DTBZ PET. PLoS One 2013;8(9):e75952.

38. Koeppe RA, Gilman S, Junck L, et al. Differentiating Alzheimer's disease from dementia with Lewy bodies and Parkinson's disease with (+)-[11C]dihydrotetrabenazine positron emission tomography. Alzheimers Dement 2008;4(1 Suppl 1): S67–76.

39. Lin SC, Lin KJ, Hsiao IT, et al. In vivo detection of monoaminergic degeneration in early Parkinson disease by (18)F-9-fluoropropyl-(+)-dihydrotetrabenazine PET. J Nucl Med 2014;55(1):73–9.

40. Bohnen NI, Albin RL, Koeppe RA, et al. Positron emission tomography of monoaminergic vesicular binding in aging and Parkinson disease. J Cereb Blood Flow Metab 2006;26(9): 1198–212.

41. Brooks DJ, Ibanez V, Sawle GV, et al. Striatal D2 receptor status in patients with Parkinson's disease, striatonigral degeneration, and progressive supranuclear palsy, measured with 11C-raclopride and positron emission tomography. Ann Neurol 1992; 31(2):184–92.

42. Singhal T, Narayanan TK, Jain V, et al. 11C-L-methionine positron emission tomography in the clinical management of cerebral gliomas. Mol Imaging Biol 2008;10(1):1–18.

43. Ishiwata K, Kubota K, Murakami M, et al. Re-evaluation of amino acid PET studies: can the protein synthesis rates in brain and tumor tissues be measured in vivo? J Nucl Med 1993;34(11):1936–43.

44. Kato T, Shinoda J, Oka N, et al. Analysis of 11C-methionine uptake in low-grade gliomas and correlation with proliferative activity. AJNR Am J Neuroradiol 2008;29(10):1867–71.

45. Herholz K, Holzer T, Bauer B, et al. 11C-methionine PET for differential diagnosis of low-grade gliomas. Neurology 1998;50:1316–22.

46. Kim CK, Alavi JB, Alavi A, et al. New grading system of cerebral gliomas using positron emission tomography with F-18 fluorodeoxyglucose. J Neurooncol 1991;10(1):85–91.

47. Spence AM, Muzi M, Mankoff DA, et al. 18F-FDG PET of gliomas at delayed intervals: improved distinction between tumor and normal gray matter. J Nucl Med 2004;45(10):1653–9.

48. Isohashi K, Shimosegawa E, Kato H, et al. Optimization of [11C]methionine PET study: appropriate scan timing and effect of plasma amino acid concentrations on the SUV. EJNMMI Res 2013;3(1):27. http://dx.doi.org/10.1186/2191-219X-3-27.

49. Herholz K, Heiss WD. Positron emission tomography in clinical neurology. Mol Imaging Biol 2004;6(4):239–69.

50. Singhal T, Narayanan TK, Jacobs MP, et al. 11C-methionine PET for grading and prognostication in gliomas: a comparison study with 18F-FDG PET and contrast enhancement on MRI. J Nucl Med 2012;53(11):1709–15.

51. Nihashi T, Dahabreh IJ, Terasawa T. Diagnostic accuracy of PET for recurrent glioma diagnosis: a meta-analysis. AJNR Am J Neuroradiol 2013;34(5):944–50 S1–11.

52. Jacobs AH, Thomas A, Kracht LW, et al. 18F-fluoro-L-thymidine and 11C-methylmethionine as markers of increased transport and proliferation in brain tumors. J Nucl Med 2005;46(12):1948–58.

53. Santambrogio L, Belyanskaya SL, Fischer FR, et al. Developmental plasticity of CNS microglia. Proc Natl Acad Sci U S A 2001;98(11):6295–300.

54. Winkeler A, Boisgard R, Martin A, et al. Radioisotopic imaging of neuroinflammation. J Nucl Med 2010;51(1):1–4.

55. Dickens AM, Vainio S, Marjamaki P, et al. Detection of microglial activation in an acute model of neuroinflammation using PET and radiotracers 11C-(R)-PK11195 and 18F-GE-180. J Nucl Med 2014;55(3):466–72.

56. Kreisl WC, Fujita M, Fujimura Y, et al. Comparison of [(11)C]-(R)-PK 11195 and [(11)C]PBR28, two radioligands for translocator protein (18 kDa) in human and monkey: implications for positron emission tomographic imaging of this inflammation biomarker. Neuroimage 2010;49(4):2924–32.

57. Kreisl WC, Jenko KJ, Hines CS, et al. A genetic polymorphism for translocator protein 18 kDa affects both in vitro and in vivo radioligand binding in human brain to this putative biomarker of neuroinflammation. J Cereb Blood Flow Metab 2013;33(1):53–8.

58. Thiel A, Radlinska BA, Paquette C, et al. The temporal dynamics of poststroke neuroinflammation: a longitudinal diffusion tensor imaging-guided PET study with 11C-PK11195 in acute subcortical stroke. J Nucl Med 2010;51(9):1404–12.

59. Giannetti P, Politis M, Su P, et al. Microglia activation in multiple sclerosis black holes predicts outcome in progressive patients: an in vivo [(11)C](R)-PK11195-PET pilot study. Neurobiol Dis 2014;65:203–10.

60. Kreisl WC, Lyoo CH, McGwier M, et al. In vivo radioligand binding to translocator protein correlates with severity of Alzheimer's disease. Brain 2013;136(Pt 7):2228–38.

61. Iannaccone S, Cerami C, Alessio M, et al. In vivo microglia activation in very early dementia with Lewy bodies, comparison with Parkinson's disease. Parkinsonism Relat Disord 2013;19(1):47–52.

62. Doorduin J, de Vries EF, Willemsen AT, et al. Neuroinflammation in schizophrenia-related psychosis: a PET study. J Nucl Med 2009;50(11):1801–7.

^{18}F-Fluoride PET/ Computed Tomography Imaging

Einat Even-Sapir, MD, PhD

KEYWORDS

- ^{18}F-fluoride • PET/CT • Computed tomography • Bone imaging

KEY POINTS

- Production of ^{18}F-labeled tracers, including ^{18}F-fluoride, has been simplified, and bone imaging using ^{18}F-fluoride PET with computed tomography (PET/CT) is relevant once again.
- ^{18}F-Fluoride PET/CT imaging should be considered for the assessment of bone abnormality in clinical practice, not only in patients with cancer but also in benign scenarios.
- Accumulated data on the use of ^{18}F-fluoride indicate that this modality is highly sensitive for the detection of skeletal lesions, allowing assessment of pathophysiologic processes in normal and abnormal bone.

INTRODUCTION

^{18}F-Fluoride, a bone-seeking PET tracer, was approved in the United States for imaging in 1972, but its clinical use lapsed because of the limited number of cyclotrons and PET systems.[1,2] In addition, in the mid-1970s ^{99m}Tc-diphosphonates were widely available and became the preferred tracer used in routine practice for scintigraphic assessment of bone abnormality.[3]

However, changes have come about. The global storage of molybdenum is now limited, affecting the availability of the ^{99m}Tc-based tracers.[4] By contrast, the number of PET/CT systems is continuously increasing, as is the number of cyclotrons and PET procedures. PET in combination with computed tomography (PET/CT) imaging has been introduced in the imaging algorithm of various clinical scenarios. Production of ^{18}F-labeled tracer including ^{18}F-fluoride has been simplified, and ^{18}F-fluoride PET/CT bone imaging is relevant once again.[3]

MECHANISM OF UPTAKE OF ^{18}F-FLUORIDE IN BONE: WHICH BONE LESIONS ACCUMULATE ^{18}F-FLUORIDE?

The uptake mechanism of ^{18}F-fluoride resembles that of ^{99m}Tc-methylene diphosphonate (MDP) but with superior pharmacokinetic characteristics. ^{18}F-Fluoride diffuses through the bone capillaries into the bone extracellular fluid (ECF) with plasma clearance more rapid than that of ^{99m}Tc-MDP, reflecting its smaller molecular weight and negligible protein binding compared with the binding of ^{99m}Tc-MDP to plasma proteins, which varies from 25% after injection to 70% 12 hours after injection.[5–7] ^{18}F-Fluoride ion exchanges with hydroxyl groups on hydroxyapatite to form fluoroapatite, and subsequently incorporated into bone matrix.[8] Correlating ^{18}F-fluoride data with CT morphology using PET/CT technology, it was reported that occasionally bone lesions that appear predominantly lytic or lucent on CT, such as lytic-type metastases and some types of bone

Department of Nuclear Medicine, Tel-Aviv Sourasky Medical Center, Sackler Faculty of Medicine, Tel-Aviv University, 6 Weizman Street, Tel-Aviv 64239, Israel
E-mail address: evensap@tlvmc.gov.il

PET Clin 9 (2014) 277–285
http://dx.doi.org/10.1016/j.cpet.2014.03.003
1556-8598/14/$ – see front matter © 2014 Elsevier Inc. All rights reserved.

cysts, may also be identified by ^{18}F-fluoride, suggesting the presence of some degree of osteoblastic activity too subtle to be appreciated morphologically, but sufficient for detection by the sensitive ^{18}F-fluoride PET.[9-13] However, it should be borne in mind that the high diagnostic performance of ^{18}F-fluoride PET is primarily in detecting bone lesions characterized by high flow and bone turnover.[2,8,9]

^{18}F-FLUORIDE PET/CT IMAGING TECHNIQUE

Patients should be well hydrated to promote rapid excretion of tracer so as to decrease the radiation dose and improve image quality. ^{18}F-Fluoride is injected intravenously, 185 to 370 MBq (5–10 mCi) in adults and 2.22 MBq/kg (0.06 mCi/kg) in children. Injection of dose in the lower range is highly suggested in young patients referred for nononcologic indications.

PET/CT acquisition can take place from 30 minutes to 4 hours after injection. In most patients, acquisition is started as early as 30 to 45 minutes after injection. However, in patients with impaired renal function or obese patients, or when the organs of interest are the extremities, delayed acquisition 90 to 120 minutes after injection may be more appropriate for better PET image quality.[14]

There are different options regarding the acquisition protocol of CT. It can be a full-dose CT; reduced-dose CT limited to a selected body region according to the clinical issue or PET findings; or CT of a larger field of view. PET can also be acquired without any CT.[15]

In PET/CT technology, CT is intended not only to provide morphologic data but also for attenuation correction. Whether there is a need for attenuation correction in the case of ^{18}F-fluoride PET is a question addressed previously by several investigators. On calculating the bone-to-muscle ratios for ^{18}F-fluoride PET images with and without attenuation correction, it has been suggested that attenuation correction is not necessary for accurate visual interpretation of ^{18}F-fluoride PET images.[16] At times, attenuation correction may eliminate PET artifacts. High tracer uptake in the renal collecting systems, for instance, was shown in young adults with back pain to interfere with assessment of the nearby spine, whereas attenuation-corrected data eliminated these artifacts. Correction, however, can be applied retrospectively if the PET data is reviewed before moving the patient from the system table.[17] It has been shown in previous studies that combining PET findings with the morphologic appearance of the lesion on CT improves specificity and leads to correct final diagnosis. The

author performs a CT with a field of view similar to that of PET using a reduced-dose CT protocol of 140 kV, 80 mA, 0.8 seconds per CT rotation, a pitch of 6, and a table speed of 22.5 mm/s, without specific breath-holding instructions. Acquisition of PET is carried out immediately following acquisition of CT, without changing the patient's positioning. Five to 9 bed positions are performed with an acquisition time of 2 to 5 minutes per bed depending on the injected activity, time from injection, body mass index, and skeletal region, whether axial or peripheral. If the indication for study is to search for metastases, similar to ^{18}F-fluorodeoxyglucose PET/CT, the author images the skeleton from skull to femurs unless lesions are suspected to be located at the distal peripheral bones; acquisition then also includes these areas. For nononcologic indications, if clinical data suggest abnormality in the peripheral skeleton, mainly the legs, PET/CT of the axial skeleton is performed with another acquisition for the legs with a longer time per bed.[11,14,18,19]

RADIATION EXPOSURE OF ^{18}F-FLUORIDE PET/CT

Injection of 185 MBq (5 mCi) ^{18}F-fluoride in adult patients is associated with an effective dose of 4.25 mGy, comparable with 4.75 mGy when 740 MBq (20 mCi) of ^{99m}Tc-MDP is injected. In children, using an administered activity of 0.055 mCi/kg (2.1 MBq/kg) was calculated to result in an effective dose that ranges from 0.31 rem (3.1 mSv) in a 1-year-old to 0.35 rem (3.5 mSv) in a 15-year-old. The target organ is the bladder.[17,20-22]

Radiation exposure of the CT portion depends on the acquisition protocol and size of the area scanned. Performing CT of the same areas as PET using a reduced-dose protocol, radiation exposure from the CT part of the study is 7.3 mGy in adults.[21]

NORMAL DISTRIBUTION OF ^{18}F-FLUORIDE

There is a large variability in the normal uptake values of ^{18}F-fluoride in different skeletal regions. The highest values are found in trabecular bones, such as in the vertebrae, characterized by greater bone turnover in comparison with long bones of the peripheral skeleton, which are predominately cortical.[23-25] In children and adolescents, uptake is increased in the metaphyses.

If renal function is intact, the kidneys and urinary bladder are visible, though not in the background soft tissue. As in the case of ^{99m}Tc-MDP bone scintigraphy, physiologic ^{18}F-fluoride uptake in the skeleton is uniform and symmetric (**Fig. 1**) and, as a rule of thumb, uptake that is higher or lower than in adjacent bone or contralateral side should be further assessed.[14] Nevertheless, in view of the high sensitivity of 18F-fluoride some inherent inhomogeneity and asymmetry can be normal more often than with routine bone scintigraphy, mainly in older patients, and reviewers should build their own experience in reading these studies and ensure to review the imaging data while considering the patient's age and clinical presentation. Determining the morphologic appearance of a suspected PET lesion by reviewing the CT may, at times, assist in differentiating a true bone abnormality from normal variation in uptake.

BENIGN INDICATIONS FOR 18F-FLUORIDE PET IMAGING

Clinical data on the use of 18F-fluoride PET/CT for benign clinical scenarios is being accumulated. Reported studies are those of visual assessment of 18F-fluoride accumulation for identification of bone abnormality, and studies in which quantification of 18F-fluoride is taking place to investigate the pathophysiologic processes occurring in normal and abnormal bone, using compartmental analysis or semiquantitative measurement of standard uptake values (SUVs).

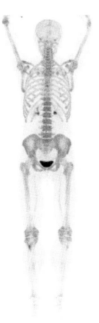

Fig. 1. 18F-Fluoride PET/CT (maximum-intensity projection) normal tracer distribution with uniform and symmetric tracer uptake in the skeleton. (*Courtesy of Mohsen Beheshti, MD, FEBNM, FASNC, PET-CT Center, Linz, Austria.*)

Various skeletal regions fall within the scope of investigation. In the skull, 18F-fluoride uptake was assessed in hyperostosis cranialis interna (HCI), a hereditary bone disease characterized by endosteal hyperostosis and osteosclerosis of the skull and skull base. In these patients, bone overgrowth causes entrapment and dysfunction of several cranial nerves. 18F-Fluoride in different skull regions measured by SUVs was assessed in 9 patients with HCI, 7 nonaffected family members and 9 non-HCI nonfamily members. Uptake was higher in the sphenoid bone and clivus regions of affected family members. Visual assessment was helpful in determining disease severity.[26] In another study on condylar hyperplasia characterized by an overgrowth of one mandibular condyle resulting in facial asymmetry, 18F-fluoride imaging was found to be valuable in differentiating active growth from nonactive growth, and had a direct impact on therapeutic approach, as high condylectomy is usually the treatment of choice in patients with active growth whereas others are managed with orthodontic treatment and orthognathic surgery.[27]

Excessive pressure caused by wearing maladaptive dentures is a cause for bone resorption beneath the denture. Using 18F-fluoride imaging, changes in bone metabolism occurring underneath the dentures were identified while not being appreciated on radiography. It has been found that in cases of well-adapted denture the bone metabolism is increased initially, decreasing at 4 months.[28]

Incidence of osteonecrosis of the jaw is increasing in view of the introduction of bisphosphonate treatment in patients with osteoporosis, Paget disease of bone, osteolytic bone metastases, and osteolytic lesions of multiple myeloma. Osteonecrosis of the jaws is a serious complication in a subset of patients receiving these drugs, leading in severe cases to exposed necrotic bone, severe pain, infection, pathologic fractures, extraoral fistula, and lysis extending to the inferior border. Early diagnosis and assessment of severity is crucial. 18F-Fluoride PET seemed to be more sensitive than 18F-FDG in detecting this abnormality, although the latter was better for monitoring response to therapy.[29,30]

Quantitative 18F-fluoride PET imaging has also been used also to assess the perfusion and osteoblastic activity of revascularized fibular grafts for mandibular reconstruction, and was found to be valuable in differentiating uneventful graft healing, early failure, and nonunion.[31–33]

In the vertebral column and pelvic bones, several articles have addressed the role of 18F-fluoride PET in patients with back pain, with or without previous back surgery. Performing ^{18}F-fluoride imaging in children and young adults with back pain,[17,34] pain was found to be related to pars defects or pedicle fracture (**Fig. 2**), trauma, sacroiliac joint inflammation, or stress fracture (**Figs. 3** and **4**), and benign tumors such as osteoid osteoma (**Fig. 5**). Of note was the high negative predictive value of a normal study, as patients who had a negative ^{18}F-fluoride PET/CT did not need any medical intervention, and the pain resolved spontaneously.[34] In a study on the use of ^{18}F-fluoride PET/CT in 67 patients with low back pain including 25 patients after fusion surgery or laminectomy, accumulation of ^{18}F-fluoride in the spine was identified in 84% of the patients, facet joint uptake being the most common site of abnormality (**Figs. 6** and **7**). One-third of the patients had both facet joints and disc lesions. ^{18}F-Fluoride PET/CT revealed vertebral abnormalities in all patients after fusion surgery and in 65%

patients presenting with pain after laminectomy.[35] ^{18}F-Fluoride PET/CT was also used to assess the natural history of what appears to be a successful incorporation of cages at intercorporeal fusion of the cervical and lumbar spine. The investigators found that increased ^{18}F-fluoride uptake can be seen in eventually successful cervical cages older than 1 year and up to almost 8 years, and up to 10 years in lumbar cages, possibly indicating stress or microinstability.[36] In the sacroiliac joints (SIJ), uptake of ^{18}F-fluoride was determined in 15 patients with active ankylosing spondylitis (AS) in a comparison with uptake in 13 control patients with mechanical low back pain. Uptake was higher in the former and was related to severity.[37] The same investigators found no full agreement between increased uptake of ^{18}F-fluoride in the vertebrae and SIJ and the presence of bone marrow edema detected on magnetic resonance (MR) imaging in patients with active AS, concluding that increased ^{18}F-fluoride uptake on PET/CT and bone marrow edema on MR imaging

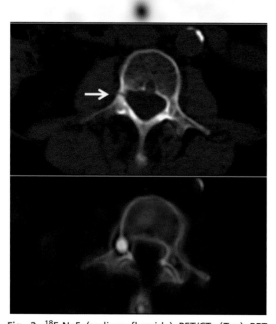

Fig. 2. ^{18}F-NaF (sodium fluoride) PET/CT. (*Top*) PET, (*middle*) CT, (*bottom*) fusion PET/CT. Focal increased tracer uptake on L3 (*top, arrow*) correlated with pedicle fracture on CT (*middle, arrow*). (*Courtesy of Mohsen Beheshti, MD, FEBNM, FASNC, PET-CT Center, Linz, Austria.*)

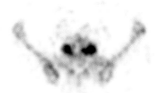

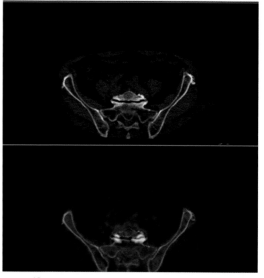

Fig. 3. ^{18}F-NaF PET/CT. (*Top*) PET, (*middle*) CT, (*bottom*) fusion PET/CT. Increased tracer uptake on sacrum (*top*) correlated with fracture on CT (*middle*). (*Courtesy of Mohsen Beheshti, MD, FEBNM, FASNC, PET-CT Center, Linz, Austria.*)

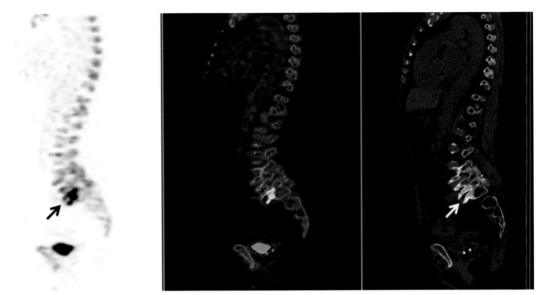

Fig. 4. ¹⁸F-NaF PET/CT. (*Left*) PET, (*middle*) fusion PET/CT, (*right*) CT. Increased tracer uptake on L4-5 (*left, arrow*) correlated with insufficiency fracture on CT (*right, arrow*). (*Courtesy of* Mohsen Beheshti, MD, FEBNM, FASNC, PET-CT Center, Linz, Austria.)

suggest different aspects of bone involvement in this condition.[38]

At the hip joint area, quantitative ¹⁸F-fluoride PET was found to be valuable for in vivo assessment of the regional blood supply of the femoral head, in addition to monitoring the changes over time and predicting of outcome in patients with osteonecrosis of the femoral head.[39] In another study, prolonged increased ¹⁸F-fluoride uptake in bone was described after hip augmentation

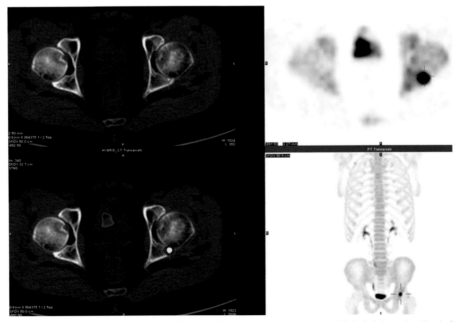

Fig. 5. ¹⁸F-Fluoride PET/CT data from a 32-year-old male patient presenting with left hip pain. The left upper image is transaxial CT of the hip area, the right upper image is PET, the left bottom image is fused PET/CT, and the right bottom image is a maximum-intensity projection of ¹⁸F-fluoride PET. Focal increased uptake is noted in the posterior aspect of the left acetabulum, corresponding in location to a focal hyperdense lesion. The final diagnosis is osteoid osteoma. (*Courtesy of* Mohsen Beheshti, MD, FEBNM, FASNC, PET-CT Center, Linz, Austria.)

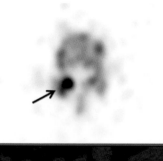

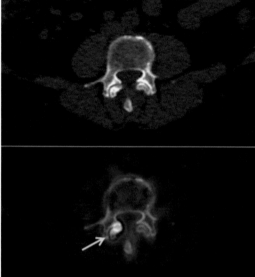

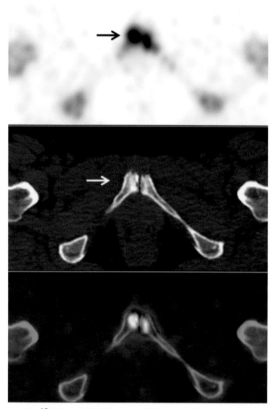

Fig. 6. ^{18}F-NaF PET/CT. (*Top*) PET, (*middle*) CT, (*bottom*) fusion PET/CT. Increased tracer uptake in right part of lumbar vertebra (*top, arrow*) is localized on right facet joint (*bottom, arrow*), suggesting facet joint arthritis. (*Courtesy of* Mohsen Beheshti, MD, FEBNM, FASNC, PET-CT Center, Linz, Austria.)

Fig. 7. ^{18}F-NaF PET/CT. (*Top*) PET, (*middle*) CT, (*bottom*) fusion PET/CT. Focal increased tracer uptake on symphysis pubis (*arrows*) suggests pubic symphysitis. (*Courtesy of* Mohsen Beheshti, MD, FEBNM, FASNC, PET-CT Center, Linz, Austria.)

surgery with allogenic acetabular grafts, compared with genuine cortical bone. It was suggested that the increased bone metabolism in allogenic bone graft is caused by reduced ability to respond to elevated metabolic demands after surgery, with continuous stress to the normal surrounding bone, and corresponding histopathologic findings of prolonged new bone formation in peripheral areas.[40] ^{18}F-Fluoride imaging was also used to assess bone remodeling in cases of osteolytic acetabular defects occurring after hip arthroplasty, and to monitor to monitor healing of morselized bone allografts after revision arthroplasty. ^{18}F-Fluoride uptake was highly elevated preoperatively in the osteolytic areas, indicating that despite predominant loss of bone, new bone formation is present at the same time. After revision, uptake increases continuously, and at 1 year after surgery declines to that of the reference contralateral bone.[41]

In the lower extremities, ^{18}F-fluoride PET/CT performed in 28 patients with unclear foot pain identified lesions that potentially could be the cause for pain that were not always identified on MR imaging, including an active os trigonum, an active nonunion after a distal tibial fracture, plantar fasciitis, subtalar osteoarthritis, an active os tibiale externum, an active neoarticulation between metatarsal bone, and osteoarthritis of metatarsophalangeal joints. It is noteworthy that abnormal findings found on ^{18}F-fluoride imaging had a direct impact on patient management, including the decision to operate.[42]

Patients who underwent anterior cruciate ligament reconstruction in the knee region, by incorporation of a tendon graft in a bone tunnel, were assessed with quantitative ^{18}F-fluoride PET to follow the regional bone turnover starting 1 day after surgery until 22 months later. Highest uptake was found 3 weeks after surgery, but the activity at the femoral fixation points was markedly increased even after 7 months. Bone turnover was almost normalized 22 months after the operation.[43]

Several publications have reported on the kinetics of ¹⁸F-fluoride uptake in metabolic bone conditions. In postmenopausal women, findings of quantitative ¹⁸F-fluoride imaging revealed that in osteoporotic patients, the global skeletal bone turnover is increased while the regional bone formation at the lumbar spine, composed of predominately trabecular bone, is reduced.[44] Quantitative assessment of the regional differences in ¹⁸F-fluoride kinetics between lumbar vertebrae and the humerus in postmenopausal women allowed a better understanding of the differences in the pathophysiology of metabolic impairment in different skeletal regions consisting of different bone type, and their response to treatment.[25] Quantitation of ¹⁸F-fluoride uptake was also found to be valuable in monitoring response to antiresorptive treatment in osteoporotic patients. After successful risedronate therapy, there was an increase in the reverse transfer of ¹⁸F-fluoride from the bone ECF to the blood and a decrease in the fraction of tracer found in the ECF, which undergoes specific binding to the bone matrix.[24]

When performed in patients with Paget disease, involved bones were characterized by increased plasma clearance of the tracer to bone, increased regional bone formation, and a tight binding of the tracer to bone. ¹⁸F-Fluoride assessment was also suggested for monitoring the response of bisphosphonate therapy in patients with Paget disease to differentiate between responders and nonresponders. Decrease in the clearance of ¹⁸F-fluoride from blood to bone was noted, although mineralization remained unaffected. Uptake was found to decrease with time, reaching normal uptake values at 6 months after successful therapy. Nonresponse was associated with an increase in SUV.[45,46]

Child abuse is an important problem whereby ¹⁸F-fluoride imaging was found to be of clinical relevance. The number of fractures and the extent of injury are often crucial in determining that abuse, as opposed to accidental injury, has occurred. Certain patterns of the distribution of fractures, the type of fractures, and the presence of fractures in locations not consistent with the reported injury are highly suggestive of child abuse. Radiographic skeletal survey remains the initial imaging modality of choice for the evaluation of fractures in cases of suspected child abuse. Nevertheless, fractures of the ribs, which are the most common location of fractures in young abused children, are overlooked initially and may be apparent on follow-up radiographs only.

Comparing the sensitivity of skeletal survey and ¹⁸F-fluoride PET for the detection of fractures in various skeletal regions in children younger than 2 years suspected of being abused, the former was found to be more sensitive for the detection of fractures in general and detection of fractures around the rib cage in particular.[47]

Recently, ¹⁸F-fluoride PET/CT was suggested also for nonosseous benign indications, such as the assessment of atherosclerotic plaques. The clinical importance of imaging in this condition is through identification of vulnerable atherosclerotic plaques that are prone to rupture. Various pathophysiologic processes are involved in the formation of plaques, including inflammation, apoptosis, and mineralization, each being a target for imaging. ¹⁸F-FDG PET may be adequate for the assessment of vascular macrophage activity, ¹⁸F-fluoride PET for the detection of active mineral deposition, and CT for the assessment of arterial calcification. Comparing the accumulation of the 2 PET tracers, one can differentiate between atherosclerotic lesions with predominant inflammation and those with predominant mineral deposition reflecting a more advanced disease. Comparing ¹⁸F-fluoride uptake with arterial calcification seen on CT, colocalization of ¹⁸F-fluoride uptake with calcification was found in most lesions (88%), whereas only one-fifth of all calcified lesions detected by CT show increased ¹⁸F-fluoride uptake, suggesting that ¹⁸F-fluoride accumulation indicates progressive disease with continuing mineral deposition, whereas plaques without ¹⁸F-fluoride uptake represent nonprogressive disease.[48,49]

SUMMARY

In view of the increasing number of cyclotrons and PET/CT systems, ¹⁸F-fluoride PET/CT imaging should be considered for the assessment of bone abnormality in clinical practice, not only in patients with cancer but also in benign scenarios. Accumulated data on the use of ¹⁸F-fluoride indicate that this modality is highly sensitive for the detection of skeletal lesions, allowing assessment of pathophysiologic processes in normal and abnormal bone.

REFERENCES

1. Blau M, Nagler W, Bender MA. A new isotope for bone scanning. J Nucl Med 1962;3:332–4.
2. Blau M, Ganatra R, Bender MA. ¹⁸F-fluoride for bone imaging. Semin Nucl Med 1972;2:31–7.
3. Grant FD, Fahey FH, Packard AB, et al. Skeletal PET with ¹⁸F-fluoride: applying new technology to an old tracer. J Nucl Med 2008;49(1):68–78.

4. Gould P. Medical isotope shortage reaches crisis level. Nature 2009;460(7253):312–3.

5. Blake GM, Park-Holoan SJ, Cook GJR, et al. Quantitative studies of bone with the use of F18-fluoride and Tc99m-methylene diphosphonate. Semin Nucl Med 2001;1:28–49.

6. Wootton R, Dore C. The single-passage extraction of ^{18}F in rabbit bone. Clin Phys Physiol Meas 1986;7: 333–43.

7. Hoh CK, Hawkins RA, Dahlbom M, et al. Whole body skeletal imaging with (^{18}F) fluoride ion and PET. J Comput Assist Tomogr 1993;17:34–41.

8. Narita N, Kato K, Nakagaki H, et al. Distribution of fluoride concentration in the rat's bone. Calcif Tissue Int 1990;46:200–4.

9. Toegel S, Hoffmann O, Wadsak W, et al. Uptake of bone-seekers is solely associated with mineralization. A study with ^{99m}Tc-MDP, [153]Sm-EDTMP and ^{18}F-fluoride on osteoblasts. Eur J Nucl Med Mol Imaging 2006;33:491–4.

10. Ishiguro K, Nakagaki H, Tsuboi S, et al. Distribution of fluoride in cortical bone of human rib. Calcif Tissue Int 1993;52:278–82.

11. Even-Sapir E, Metser U, Flusser G, et al. Assessment of malignant skeletal disease with ^{18}F-fluoride PET/CT. J Nucl Med 2004;45:272–8.

12. Kawaguchi M, Tateishi U, Shizukuishi K, et al. ^{18}F-fluoride uptake in bone metastasis: morphologic and metabolic analysis on integrated PET/CT. Ann Nucl Med 2010;24(4):241–7.

13. Hsu WK, Virk MS, Feeley BT, et al. Characterization of osteolytic, osteoblastic, and mixed lesions in a prostate cancer mouse model using ^{18}F-FDG and ^{18}F-fluoride PET/CT. J Nucl Med 2008;49(3):414–21.

14. Segall G, Delbeke D, Stabin MG, et al. SNM practice guideline for sodium ^{18}F-fluoride PET/CT bone scans 1.0. J Nucl Med 2010;51(11):1813–20.

15. Huang B, Law MW, Khong PL. Whole-body PET/CT scanning: estimation of radiation dose and cancer risk. Radiology 2009;251(1):166–74.

16. Tayama Y, Takahashi N, Oka T, et al. Clinical evaluation of the effect of attenuation correction technique on ^{18}F-fluoride PET images. Ann Nucl Med 2007;21: 93–9.

17. Lim R, Fahey FH, Drubach LA, et al. Early experience with fluorine-18 sodium fluoride bone PET in young patients with back pain. J Pediatr Orthop 2007;27:277–82.

18. Even-Sapir E, Metser U, Mishani E, et al. The detection of bone metastases in patients with high-risk prostate cancer: [99m]Tc- MDP planar BS, single- and multi-field-of-view SPECT, ^{18}F-fluoride PET, and ^{18}F-fluoride PET/CT. J Nucl Med 2006;47:287–97.

19. Even-Sapir E, Mishani E, Flusser G, et al. ^{18}F-fluoride positron emission tomography and positron emission tomography/computed tomography. Semin Nucl Med 2007;37:462–9.

20. Brix G, Lechel U, Glatting G, et al. Radiation exposure of patients undergoing whole-body dual-modality ^{18}F-FDG PET/CT examinations. J Nucl Med 2005;46:608–13.

21. Fahey FH, Palmer MR, Strauss KJ, et al. Dosimetry and adequacy of CT-based attenuation correction for pediatric PET: phantom study. Radiology 2007; 243:96–104.

22. Gelfand MJ. Dosimetry of FDG PET/CT and other molecular imaging applications in pediatric patients. Pediatr Radiol 2009;39(Suppl 1):S46–56.

23. Schiepers C, Nuyts J, Bormans G, et al. Fluoride kinetics of the axial skeleton measured in vivo with fluorine-18-fluoride PET. J Nucl Med 1997;38:1970–6.

24. Frost ML, Cook GJ, Blake GM, et al. A prospective study of risedronate on regional bone metabolism and blood flow at the lumbar spine measured by ^{18}F-fluoride positron emission tomography. J Bone Miner Res 2003;18:2215–22.

25. Cook GJ, Lodge MA, Blake GM, et al. Differences in skeletal kinetics between vertebral and humeral bone measured by ^{18}F-fluoride positron emission tomography in postmenopausal women. J Bone Miner Res 2000;15:763–9.

26. Waterval JJ, Van Dongen TM, Stokroos RJ, et al. Bone metabolic activity in hyperostosis cranialis interna measured with ^{18}F-fluoride PET. Eur J Nucl Med Mol Imaging 2011;38(5):884–93.

27. Laverick S, Bounds G, Wong WL. [^{18}F]-fluoride positron emission tomography for imaging condylar hyperplasia. Br J Oral Maxillofac Surg 2009;47(3): 196–9.

28. Suenaga H, Yokoyama M, Yamaguchi K, et al. Time course of bone metabolism at the residual ridge beneath dentures observed using ^{18}F-fluoride positron emission computerized-tomography/computed tomography (PET/CT). Ann Nucl Med 2012;26(10): 817–22.

29. Raje N, Woo SB, Hande K, et al. Clinical, radiographic, and biochemical characterization of multiple myeloma patients with osteonecrosis of the jaw. Clin Cancer Res 2008;14(8):2387–95.

30. Wilde F, Steinhoff K, Frerich B, et al. Positron-emission tomography imaging in the diagnosis of bisphosphonate-related osteonecrosis of the jaw. Oral Surg Oral Med Oral Pathol Oral Radiol Endod 2009;107(3):412–9.

31. Schliephake H, Berding G, Knapp WH, et al. Monitoring of graft perfusion and osteoblast activity in revascularised fibula segments using [^{18}F]-positron emission tomography. Int J Oral Maxillofac Surg 1999;28:349–55.

32. Berding G, Burchert W, van den Hoff J, et al. Evaluation of the incorporation of bone grafts used in maxillofacial surgery with [^{18}F]fluoride ion and dynamic positron emission tomography. Eur J Nucl Med 1995;22:1133–40.

33. Berding G, Schliephake H, van den Hoff J, et al. Assessment of the incorporation of revascularized fibula grafts used for mandibular reconstruction with F-18-PET. Nuklearmedizin 2001;40:51–8.

34. Ovadia D, Metser U, Lievshitz G, et al. Back pain in adolescents: assessment with integrated ^{18}F-fluoride positron-emission tomography-computed tomography. J Pediatr Orthop 2007;27:90–3.

35. Gamie S, El-Maghraby T. The role of PET/CT in evaluation of facet and disc abnormalities in patients with low back pain using (18)F-fluoride. Nucl Med Rev Cent East Eur 2008;11(1):17–21.

36. Fischer DR, Zweifel K, Treyer V, et al. Assessment of successful incorporation of cages after cervical or lumbar intercorporeal fusion with [(18)F]fluoride positron-emission tomography/computed tomography. Eur Spine J 2011;20(4):640–8.

37. Strobel K, Fischer DR, Tamborrini G, et al. ^{18}F-fluoride PET/CT for detection of sacroiliitis in ankylosing spondylitis (AS). Eur J Nucl Med Mol Imaging 2010; 37(9):1760–5.

38. Fischer DR, Pfirrmann CW, Zubler V, et al. High bone turnover assessed by [18]F -fluoride PET/CT in the spine and sacroiliac joints (SIJ) of patients with ankylosing spondylitis (AS): comparison with inflammatory lesions detected by whole body MRI. EJNMMI Res 2012;2(1):38.

39. Schiepers C, Broos P, Miserez M, et al. Measurement of skeletal flow with positron emission tomography and ^{18}F-fluoride in femoral head osteonecrosis. Arch Orthop Trauma Surg 1998;118:131–5.

40. Piert M, Winter E, Becker GA, et al. Allogenic bone graft viability after hip revision arthroplasty assessed by dynamic [^{18}F]fluoride ion positron emission tomography. Eur J Nucl Med 1999;26:615–24.

41. Ullmark G, Sörensen J, Nilsson O. Bone healing of severe acetabular defects after revision arthroplasty. Acta Orthop 2009;80(2):179–83.

42. Fischer DR, Maquieira GJ, Espinosa N, et al. Therapeutic impact of [(18)F]fluoride positron-emission tomography/computed tomography on patients with unclear foot pain. Skeletal Radiol 2010;39(10):987–97.

43. Sörensen J, Michaelsson K, Strand H, et al. Longstanding increased bone turnover at the fixation points after anterior cruciate ligament reconstruction: a positron emission tomography (PET) study of 8 patients. Acta Orthop 2006;77:921–5.

44. Frost ML, Fogelman I, Blake GM, et al. Dissociation between global markers of bone formation and direct measurement of spinal bone formation in osteoporosis. J Bone Miner Res 2004;19:1797–804.

45. Cook GJ, Blake GM, Marsden PK, et al. Quantification of skeletal kinetic indices in Paget's disease using dynamic ^{18}F-fluoride positron emission tomography. J Bone Miner Res 2002;17:854–9.

46. Installé J, Nzeusseu A, Bol A, et al. (18)F-fluoride PET for monitoring therapeutic response in Paget's disease of bone. J Nucl Med 2005;46:1650–8.

47. Drubach LA, Johnston PR, Newton AW, et al. Skeletal trauma in child abuse: detection with ^{18}F-NaF PET. Radiology 2010;255(1):173–81.

48. Derlin T, Richter U, Bannas P, et al. Feasibility of ^{18}F-sodium fluoride PET/CT for imaging of atherosclerotic plaque. J Nucl Med 2010;51(6):862–5.

49. Derlin T, Tóth Z, Papp L, et al. Correlation of inflammation assessed by ^{18}F-FDG PET, active mineral deposition assessed by ^{18}F-fluoride PET, and vascular calcification in atherosclerotic plaque: a dual-tracer PET/CT study. J Nucl Med 2011;52(7):1020–7.

^{18}F-Fluoride PET and PET/CT in Children and Young Adults

Frederick D. Grant, MD*

KEYWORDS

- ^{18}F-fluoride PET • ^{18}F-fluoride PET/CT • Pediatrics • Children • Back pain • Child abuse
- Benign skeletal lesions • Pediatric musculoskeletal tumors

KEY POINTS

- In children and young adults, ^{18}F-fluoride PET and PET/computed tomography (CT) is used primarily to evaluate nonmalignant disease.
- One of the most common indications for ^{18}F-fluoride PET and PET/CT in children and young adults is back pain.
- ^{18}F-fluoride PET/CT is particularly useful for evaluating back pain in athletes and dancers, patients with scoliosis, after trauma, or in the setting of prior back surgery.
- In the evaluation of possible child abuse, ^{18}F-fluoride PET/CT is more sensitive than radiographic bone survey for detecting skeletal lesion in the chest, including ribs, spine, clavicles, scapulae, and sternum.
- Although rarely used for identification of skeletal metastases in children, ^{18}F-fluoride PET/CT may have a future role in staging pediatric musculoskeletal tumors.

After decades of being overshadowed by ^{99m}Tc-labeled bisphosphonates, ^{18}F-sodium fluoride PET has undergone a resurgence in use for bone imaging. This likely is due primarily to the increasing availability of PET/computed tomography (CT) scanners and improved logistics for the delivery of fluorine-18–labeled radiopharmaceuticals, but also may reflect the higher-quality images that can be acquired with ^{18}F-sodium fluoride PET/CT, compared to bone scintigraphy performed with ^{99m}Tc-methylene diphosphonate (^{99m}Tc-MDP).[1] Most studies demonstrating the clinical utility of ^{18}F-fluoride PET and PET/CT have been performed in adults, and there is less experience with this technique in children and young adults. Most of these studies have focused on the use of ^{18}F-fluoride PET to identify osseous metastases in patients with malignancy. In pediatric patients, the indication

for ^{18}F-fluoride PET is less likely to be malignancy and more likely to be a benign condition.

TECHNICAL PROCEDURES

In general, the procedure for ^{18}F-fluoride PET and PET/CT in children is similar to that in adults. One difference is that infants and young children may require sedation or anesthesia to cooperate with skeletal PET with ^{18}F-fluoride, although the frequency may be little different than the need for sedation or anesthesia with single-photon emission computed tomography (SPECT) or SPECT/CT of bone performed with ^{99m}Tc-MDP.

In children, the administered activity of ^{18}F-fluoride should be adjusted for patient size, following the recommendations of the North American consensus guidelines[2,3] or European Dosage

Division of Nuclear Medicine and Molecular Imaging, Department of Radiology, Boston Children's Hospital, and The Joint Program in Nuclear Medicine, Harvard Medical School, 300 Longwood Avenue, Boston, MA 02115, USA
* Division of Nuclear Medicine and Molecular Imaging, Department of Radiology, Boston Children's Hospital, Boston, MA 02115.
E-mail address: frederick.grant@childrens.harvard.edu

PET Clin 9 (2014) 287–297
http://dx.doi.org/10.1016/j.cpet.2014.03.004
1556-8598/14/$ – see front matter © 2014 Elsevier Inc. All rights reserved.

Card.[4] For example, the North American consensus guidelines recommend a dose of 2.2 MBq/kg (0.06 mCi/kg) with a minimum dose of 18.5 MBq (0.5 mCi). Therefore, this guideline would recommend an administered activity of 154 MBq (4.2 mCi) for a patient weighing 70 kg. This may be less than activity administered to an adult patient in a typical general nuclear medicine practice, but is sufficient to provide a high-quality diagnostic study, while limiting radiation exposure. Although dose estimates may vary depending on the different models of ^{18}F-fluoride and ^{99m}Tc-MDP biokinetics,[1,5] the effective dose resulting from ^{18}F-fluoride PET is similar to that provided by an appropriate weight-based administered activity of ^{99m}Tc-MDP.[1,6]

The radiation exposure from low-dose CT performed for skeletal localization will be similar for PET/CT and SPECT/CT. Organ-specific radiation exposure and effective dose will depend on the CT parameters and the imaging field of view.[7,8] One disadvantage of ^{18}F-fluoride PET is that a CT should be acquired for attenuation correction. In an early study using ^{18}F-fluoride PET, Lim and colleagues[9] demonstrated the need for attenuation correction to limit attenuation artifacts due to tracer accumulation in the renal collecting system. This may be particularly important in pediatric nuclear medicine, where the most common indication for ^{18}F-fluoride PET is back pain and suspected benign spine disease. Alternatively, delayed imaging may minimize this type of attenuation artifact with little effect on overall skeleton-to-background uptake ratio.[10] However, with most integrated PET/CT scanners, PET cannot be performed with an attenuation CT scan. Usually, a low-dose CT will suffice for both attenuation correction and skeletal localization.

No special patient preparation is needed for ^{18}F-fluoride PET. ^{18}F-fluoride is administered intravenously through indwelling or temporary intravenous access. Patients should be encouraged to drink fluids and then to void before imaging is started. Similar to ^{99m}Tc-MDP, approximately 50% of the administered dose of ^{18}F-fluoride is taken up by bone.[11] There is minimal protein binding of ^{18}F-fluoride,[12] whereas approximately 30% of ^{99m}Tc-MDP becomes protein bound immediately after administration.[13] As a result, soft tissue clearance is much faster for ^{18}F-fluoride than for ^{99m}Tc-MDP,[14] and ^{18}F-fluoride PET can be started as soon as 30 minutes after tracer administration. However, for imaging bones in the arms and legs, it may be helpful to delay the start of extremity imaging until up to 2 hours after tracer administration.[15]

The 3-phase bone scan is an important technique in skeletal scintigraphy, especially in pediatric patients. It has not been used with ^{18}F-fluoride PET, which may, in part, reflect concerns about the feasibility of angiographic and soft tissue (blood pool) phase imaging using a radiopharmaceutical with fast soft tissue clearance. Recent reports in dogs[16] and humans[17,18] have demonstrated the feasibility of dynamic imaging to image the early soft tissue distribution of tracer with ^{18}F-fluoride PET. In adult patients with the clinical diagnosis of chronic osteomyelitis, dynamic PET was performed with list mode acquisition for the first 5 minutes after ^{18}F-fluoride administration. Significantly higher soft tissue accumulation of tracer was observed in the region of disease, compared to uninvolved sites in the contralateral limb or soft tissue uptake on the skeletal phase images.[18] This procedure has not yet been well studied, so that the clinical utility of early dynamic ^{18}F-fluoride PET has not been established.

CLINICAL INDICATIONS FOR ^{18}F-FLUORIDE PET/CT

[18]F-fluoride and ^{99m}Tc-MDP have similar patterns of osseous uptake,[19] so that the approach to interpreting ^{18}F-fluoride PET/CT is similar to ^{99m}Tc-MDP scintigraphy. As in adults, ^{18}F-fluoride PET/CT is used to identify osseous metastatic disease in pediatric patients. However, in children and young adults, ^{18}F-fluoride PET/CT is used more commonly to evaluate nonmalignant abnormalities of the skeleton. At Boston Children's Hospital, the most common indication for ^{18}F-fluoride PET/CT is back pain. In a young athlete or dancer, there may be concern for injury to the vertebral pars interarticularis. This injury must be distinguished from other causes of back pain, including degenerative changes involving the intervertebral facet joint. Back pain also can be related to stress or trauma at other sites in the axial skeleton, scoliosis, prior back surgery, or benign osseous lesions, such as osteoid osteoma. Unfortunately, child abuse remains another frequent reason for performing ^{18}F-fluoride PET/CT. Because quantitative assessment of bone uptake is possible, ^{18}F-fluoride PET/CT also can be used to quantitatively assess bone turnover in a variety of settings.

Back Pain in Children, Adolescents, and Young Adults

Evaluation of back pain is the most common indication for ^{18}F-fluoride PET/CT in children and young adults.[9,20,21] One of the most common causes of

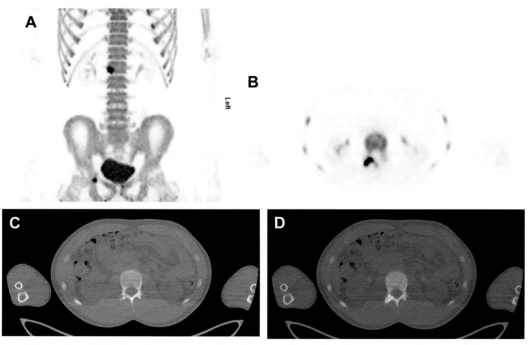

Fig. 1. 18F-fluoride PET/CT identifies pars stress in a 17-year-old male left-handed baseball pitcher who complains of right-sided low back pain that worsens with back extension. (A) A maximal intensity projection (MIP) of the lower back demonstrates intense uptake on the right side of vertebra L2. (B) Transaxial PET image shows intense uptake in the right L2 posterior elements. (C) Low-dose CT of the spine shows sclerosis in the right pars of vertebra L2. (D) Coregistration of PET and CT confirms abnormal bone turnover in the right pars interarticularis of vertebra L2. Note increased bone turnover in the left humerus of this left-handed pitcher.

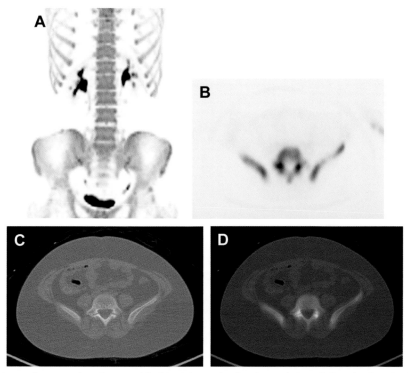

Fig. 2. Bilateral pars fractures in a 9-year-old girl with cerebral palsy and chronic low back pain. (A) An anterior projection of an MIP of the 18F-fluoride PET does not reveal abnormal uptake in the lower spine. (B) Transaxial PET image shows intense uptake in the posterior elements of vertebra L5, bilaterally. (C) Low-dose CT shows bilateral, nondisplaced fractures of the pars interarticularis of vertebra L5. (D) PET/CT fusion image confirms intense bone turnover at both sites of spondylolysis.

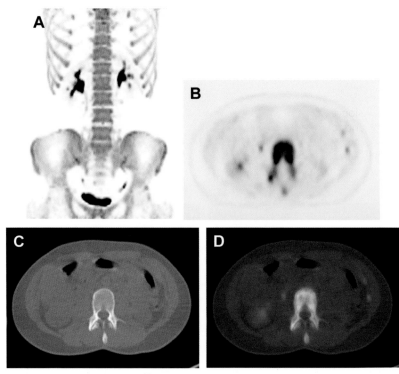

Fig. 3. Spinal facet arthropathy identified by ^{18}F-fluoride PET/CT in a 19-year-old female volleyball player with lower back pain. (A) Anterior projection of an MIP of the spine and pelvis reveals little abnormal uptake. (B) Transaxial PET slice shows intense uptake in the right posterior elements in the midlumbar spine. (C) CT shows minimal sclerosis at a right facet joint. (D) PET/CT fusion image confirms intense bone turnover at the right L3-L4 facet joint.

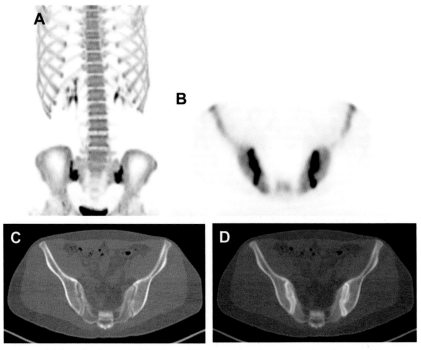

Fig. 4. Eighteen-year-old female dancer with extension-based low back pain for the past 10 months. (A) ^{18}F-fluoride PET/CT MIP shows intense uptake at both sacroiliac joints. (B) Transaxial PET slice shows intense bone turnover throughout both sacroiliac joints. (C) CT shows minimal abnormality along both sacroiliac joints. (D) PET/CT fusion image confirms intense bone turnover along both sacroiliac joints. No abnormal uptake was identified in posterior elements of the lumbar spine.

clinically significant back pain is injury to the pars interarticularis of the lumbar vertebrae in athletes and dancers.[22] Similar to ^{99m}Tc-MDP SPECT,[23] ^{18}F-fluoride PET/CT may detect increased bone turnover in a vertebral pars interarticularis as an indicator of stress injury or fracture (spondylolysis).[9] Repetitive hyperextension injury of the spine, for example in athletes and dancers, can produce stress injury or fracture of the pars interarticularis, which will result in increased bone turnover (**Fig. 1**). If there is a pars fracture, increased bone turnover will persist until the process of healing and remodeling is complete (**Fig. 2**). Bone scintigraphy with either agent provides a sensitive method for identifying bone stress injury before significant anatomic remodeling or fracture occurs. These patients may respond best to early intervention and treatment[23] without progression to fracture.

In pediatric patients with back pain, CT will show findings of pars fracture in only about half of those with abnormal focal uptake on ^{18}F-fluoride PET/CT.[1] That is, patients without CT findings may have pars stress without spondylolysis. When the ^{18}F-fluoride PET/CT is normal, CT usually will confirm the absence of a pars abnormality. However, in a small number of patients with long-standing back pain, spondylolysis identified by CT will not be associated with abnormal uptake on ^{18}F-fluoride PET/CT; this indicates little bone turnover or complete healing at the site of the prior fracture and is thought to make it unlikely that the spondylolysis is the cause of the back pain.[1]

^{18}F-fluoride PET/CT also detects abnormalities with other causes of adolescent back pain.[9,21] For example, increased bone turnover is seen at sites of facet arthropathy (**Fig. 3**). Hybrid PET/CT can be particularly helpful to distinguish pars stress and facet joint disease. Similar to ^{99m}Tc-MDP scintigraphy,[24] ^{18}F-fluoride PET/CT will identify sites of increased bone turnover at other sites of stress or traumatic injury, including the vertebral body, the spinous and transverse processes, and the sacroiliac joint (**Fig. 4**). In patients with a transitional vertebra at the lumbar sacral junction, a

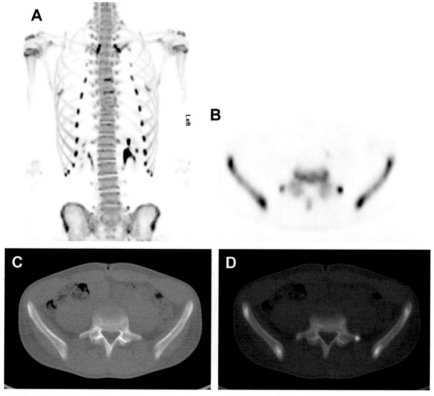

Fig. 5. ^{18}F-fluoride PET/CT identifies abnormal bone turnover related to a lumbosacral transitional vertebrae in a 14-year-old male lacrosse player. (*A*) PET MIP shows a small focus of increased uptake in the left transverse process of vertebra L5 and mildly increased uptake in the nearby sacral ala. (*B*) Transaxial PET slice shows focal ^{18}F-fluoride uptake. (*C*) CT confirms sclerosis along the transverse processes of the lowest lumbar vertebra. (*D*) PET/CT fusion image confirms increased bone turnover in the left transverse process, in close proximity to the sacral ala. This pattern of uptake suggests development of a pseudoarthrosis between the transverse process and ala.

pseudoarthrosis may develop at a site of contact between the vertebral transverse process and the sacral ala. This is characterized by increased bone turnover,[25] which can be associated with lower back pain and can be detected by ^{18}F-fluoride PET/CT (**Fig. 5**).

Scoliosis and Spinal Surgery

In patients with scoliosis or who have undergone spinal surgery, ^{18}F-fluoride PET/CT can be helpful for evaluating back pain. Patients can experience post-operative pain related to incomplete bone healing or osseous nonunion, hardware loosening, or infection. PET/CT can help localize the site of abnormal bone turnover and particularly be useful when implanted orthopedic hardware limits or prevents the use of CT or magnetic resonance imaging (MRI) to image the spine.[26] The availability of correlative CT acquired with the hybrid PET/CT can be helpful for localization of sites of abnormal bone turnover in the post-operative spine (**Fig. 6**).

However, the presence of orthopedic hardware raises concerns about attenuation artifacts, and sites of increased ^{18}F-fluoride uptake should be confirmed on PET images reconstructed without attenuation correction.

Benign Bone Lesions

[18]F-fluoride PET/CT is used to assess skeletal pain involving sites other than the spine. For example, increased bone turnover is detected at sites of stress injury or fracture in the legs and feet (**Fig. 7**). However, for these cases, ^{18}F-fluoride PET/CT may not have clear benefit over conventional bone scintigraphy. ^{18}F-fluoride PET/CT also has been reported to identify rib fractures.[21] Similar to conventional bone scintigraphy, ^{18}F-fluoride PET/CT can identify increased bone turnover at the ischiopubic synchondrosis.[21]

The high image quality of PET and the availability of hybrid CT can make ^{18}F-fluoride PET/CT very useful for localizing and characterizing other

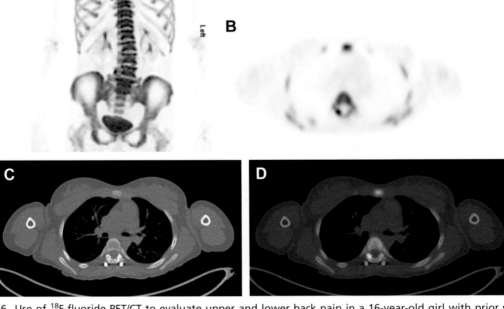

Fig. 6. Use of ^{18}F-fluoride PET/CT to evaluate upper and lower back pain in a 16-year-old girl with prior spinal fusion surgery for scoliosis. (*A*) PET MIP shows scoliosis. There is increased uptake at the site of spinal fusion in the right lumbar spine, but no abnormal uptake is identified near the site of pain in the upper back. (*B*) Transaxial PET slice shows focally increased uptake in the right posterior elements of an upper thoracic vertebra. (*C*) CT demonstrates the location of spinal orthopedic hardware, including screws attaching the rods to the spine. (*D*) Fusion images confirm increased bone turnover adjacent to an intraosseous screw near the superior end of the right-sided rod in the posterior elements of a midthoracic vertebra, probably T5. The patient's upper back symptoms improved after surgical adjustment of the orthopedic hardware.

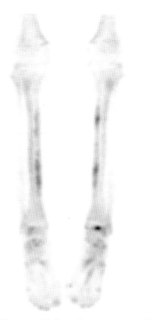

benign osseous lesions. For example, ^{18}F-fluoride PET/CT has been used in patients with suspected osteoblastoma or osteoid osteoma of either the spine or elsewhere in the skeleton (**Fig. 8**).[21,27] ^{18}F-fluoride PET/CT also can be used to identify sites of other benign osseous diseases, such as Paget disease[17] and Langerhans cell histiocytosis.

Quantitative Bone Metabolism

^{18}F-fluoride PET/CT provides a noninvasive method to quantitatively assess skeletal bone turnover that has been shown to correlate with bone histomorphometry and serum markers of bone turnover.[28,29] In adults, ^{18}F-fluoride PET has been used to assess bone turnover in patients with renal osteodystrophy,[28] Paget disease,[30] and post-menopausal osteoporosis.[31] Similar studies may be useful for research or clinical studies of bone turnover in patients with eating disorders.[32]

Bone Viability

^{18}F-fluoride PET/CT has been used to assess bone viability and healing after trauma or surgery by quantitative assessment of regional bone uptake.[33] Most of these applications have been in adults undergoing joint surgery with resurfacing arthroplasty[34] or bone grafting,[35,36] in whom ^{18}F-fluoride

Fig. 7. In a 17-year-old female runner with bilateral leg pain, ^{18}F-fluoride PET shows increased cortical uptake in both tibiae consistent with stress changes, whereas focal uptake along the posteromedial aspect of the left tibia is concerning for stress fracture. Focal uptake at the tibiotalor junctions has no radiographic correlate and likely represents stress changes.

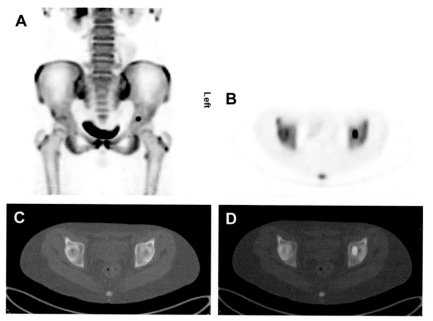

Fig. 8. Evaluation of a 14-year-old girl with groin pain that is relieved by nonsteroidal pain reliever. MRI and CT identified a sclerotic lesion in the superior aspect of the acetabulum. (*A*) ^{18}F-fluoride PET MIP shows focal uptake in the superior aspect of the left acetabulum. (*B*) Transaxial PET images show intense focal uptake in the superior aspect of the left acetabulum. (*C*) Low-dose CT shows a subchondral sclerotic lesion in left acetabulum. (*D*) PET/CT fusion images confirm that the site of intense bone turnover corresponds to the focal lesion on CT, most consistent with an osteoid osteoma.

PET was used to assess post-operative bone viability. In one small study of adults with hip fracture, decreased osseous blood flow or decreased skeletal uptake of ^{18}F-fluoride, as measured by dynamic ^{18}F-fluoride PET, predicted a future need for joint replacement surgery.[37] In patients with atraumatic osteonecrosis of the femoral head,[38] ^{18}F-fluoride PET showed increased uptake in the acetabulum of approximately half the involved joints. Additional study is needed to determine if the quantitative assessment of bone metabolism with ^{18}F-fluoride PET has clinical utility in the management of pediatric patients with femoral head avascular necrosis.

Skeletal Injury in Child Abuse

Fractures are a common finding in children with suspected child abuse. A radiographic skeletal survey is the primary method for identifying fractures,[39] while conventional bone scintigraphy has had a role as an alternate imaging study. Drubach and colleagues[40] compared the performance of skeletal survey and ^{18}F-fluoride PET in 22 children aged less than 2 years. ^{18}F-fluoride PET identified more fractures (85%) than skeletal survey (72%). ^{18}F-fluoride PET was more sensitive for identifying fractures in the thorax, including spine, ribs, clavicles, scapulae, and sternum. In particular, ^{18}F-fluoride PET detected 93% and skeletal survey detected 73% of posterior rib fractures. Although additional posterior rib fractures were identified with follow-up radiographs, ^{18}F-fluoride PET provides the additional benefit of early diagnosis, at the time clinical decisions are being made. However, for detection of classic metaphyseal lesions, more findings were detected by skeletal survey (80%) than ^{18}F-fluoride PET (67%). ^{18}F-fluoride PET without CT also has lower sensitivity than CT alone for identifying skull fractures. Therefore, full evaluation of a child with suspected abuse likely will continue to include radiographic skeletal survey complemented by bone scan, such as ^{18}F-fluoride PET/CT (**Fig. 9**).

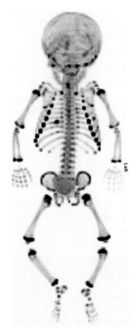

Fig. 9. Use of ^{18}F-fluoride PET/CT to evaluate a 3-month-old infant with concern for child abuse. Intense uptake in the right posterior eighth rib corresponds to a rib fracture identified on skeletal survey. Less intense uptake in the right posterior tenth, left anterolateral fifth, and left lateral seventh ribs also likely represents other rib fractures that were not detected by radiography. Focal uptake in the distal right ulna also suggests trauma or fracture.

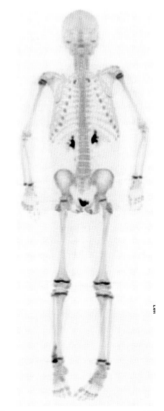

Fig. 10. ^{18}F-fluoride PET in an 8-year-old boy with Ewing sarcoma of the right fibula shows increased uptake in the primary lesion. No other sites of osseous abnormality are identified. This demonstrates the use of ^{18}F-fluoride PET to image the whole skeleton in children and young adults with musculoskeletal tumors.

Cancer Imaging

Although a less common indication in children than in adults, bone scintigraphy can have a role in identifying skeletal metastases in childhood cancers. Currently, ^{18}F-fluoride PET/CT is not used routinely for whole skeleton surveys in pediatric oncology patients. No clinical trials have been performed to demonstrate the utility of ^{18}F-fluoride PET/CT in childhood cancer. For example, it is not known if the higher sensitivity of ^{18}F-fluoride PET/CT for skeletal metastases observed in adults will translate to pediatrics.

^{18}F-fluoride PET/CT may have a role in the management of some tumors, such as osteosarcoma, for which conventional bone scintigraphy is preferred over ^{18}F-FDG PET/CT. Bone scan is a highly sensitive method of identifying the primary tumor and skeletal metastases of osteosarcoma.[41] Bone imaging also remains an important part of the evaluation of Ewing sarcoma. In some circumstances, ^{18}F-fluoride PET/CT could have role in the evaluation of skeletal disease in patients with musculoskeletal tumors (**Fig. 10**). ^{18}F-fluoride uptake also may be seen in osteoblastic pulmonary metastases of osteosarcoma. Similar to ^{99m}Tc-MDP bone scintigraphy, ^{18}F-fluoride PET/CT may demonstrate increased uptake in some soft tissues, such as neuroblastoma (**Fig. 11**).

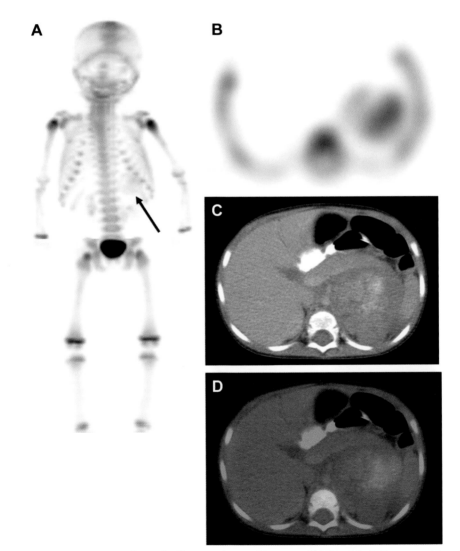

Fig. 11. In an 18-month-old girl with newly diagnosed neuroblastoma, ^{18}F-fluoride PET was used for staging. (*A*) The PET MIP shows no abnormal skeletal uptake, but abnormal tracer accumulation is seen in the upper left quadrant of the abdomen. (*B*) A transaxial PET slice confirms the location of the extra-osseous uptake. (*C*) The previous diagnostic CT demonstrates a large soft tissue suprarenal mass that contains calcifications. (*D*) Co-registration of PET and CT images confirms extra-osseous ^{18}F-fluoride uptake in the primary tumor (*arrow*).

SUMMARY

[18]F-fluoride PET/CT has been used for a wide variety of indications in children and young adults. Nearly all pediatric ^{18}F-fluoride PET/CTs are performed to evaluate benign conditions. The most common indication is the evaluation of back pain in a wide variety of circumstances, including patients with sports injuries, scoliosis, trauma, and back pain after surgery. The high image quality of ^{18}F-fluoride PET/CT can make it particularly useful for evaluating benign skeletal lesions such as osteoid osteoma and Langerhans cell histiocytosis. Quantitative assessment of bone turnover with ^{18}F-fluoride PET/CT may make it useful for assessing the skeleton in patients with metabolic bone diseases, eating disorders, and avascular necrosis. There is little pediatric experience using ^{18}F-fluoride PET/CT for evaluation of skeletal or soft tissue disease in childhood cancers.

REFERENCES

1. Grant FD, Fahey FH, Packard AG, et al. Skeletal PET with 18F-fluoride: applying new technology to an old tracer. J Nucl Med 2008;49:68–78.
2. Gelfand MJ, Parisi MT, Treves ST. Pediatric radiopharmaceutical administered doses: 2010 North American consensus guidelines. J Nucl Med 2011; 52:318–22.
3. Treves ST, Parisi MT, Gelfand MJ. Pediatric radiopharmaceutical doses: new guidelines. Radiology 2011;261:347–9.
4. Lassman M, Biassoni L, Monsieurs M, et al. The new EANM paediatric dosage card. Eur J Nucl Med Mol Imaging 2007;34:796–8.
5. Ohnona J, Michaud L, Balogova S, et al. Can we achieve a radionuclide radiation dose equal to or less than that of 99mTc-hydroxymethane diphosphonate bone scintigraphy with a low-dose 18F—sodium fluoride time-of-flight PET of diagnostic quality. Nucl Med Commun 2013;34:417–25.
6. Grant FD, Drubach LA, Treves ST, et al. Updated estimated radiation doses for paediatric nuclear medicine studies. London: International Pediatric Radiology Congress; 2011.
7. Gelfand MJ, Lemen LC. PET/CT and SPECT/CT dosimetry in children: the challenges to the pediatric imager. Semin Nucl Med 2007;37:391–8.
8. Gelfand MJ. Dose reduction in pediatric hybrid and planar imaging. Q J Nucl Med Mol Imaging 2010;54: 379–88.
9. Lim R, Fahey FH, Drubach LA, et al. Early experience with fluorine-18 sodium fluoride bone PET in young patients with back pain. J Pediatr Orthop 2007;27:277–82.
10. Kurdziel KA, Shih JH, Apolo AB, et al. The kinetics and reproducibility of 18F-sodium fluoride for oncology using current PET camera technology. J Nucl Med 2012;53:1175–84.
11. Chilton HM, Francis MD, Thrall JH. Radiopharmaceuticals for bone and bone marrow imaging. In: Swanson DP, Chilton HM, Thrall JH, editors. Pharmaceuticals in medical imaging: radioopaque contrast media, radiopharmaceuticals, enhancement agents for magnetic resonance imaging and ultrasound. New York: Macmillan Pub Co; 1990. p. 537–63.
12. Blake GM, Park-Holohan SJ, Cook GL, et al. Quantitative studies of bone with the use of 18F-fluoride and 99mTc-methylene diphosphonate. Semin Nucl Med 2001;31:28–49.
13. Hyldstrup L, McNair P, Ring P, et al. Studies on diphosphonate kinetics. Part I: evaluation of plasma elimination curves during 24 h. Eur J Nucl Med 1987;12:581–4.
14. Park-Holohan SJ, Blake GM, Fogelman I. Quantitative studies of bone with the use of 18F-fluoride and 99mTc-methylene diphosphonate: evaluation of renal and whole-blood kinetics. Nucl Med Commun 2001;22(9):1037–44.
15. Segall G, Delbeke D, Stabin MG, et al. SNM practice guideline for sodium 18F-fluoride PET/CT bone scans 1.0. J Nucl Med 2010;51:1813–20.
16. Valdés-Martínez A, Kraft SL, Brundage CM, et al. Assessment of blood pool, soft tissue, and skeletal uptake of sodium fluoride F 18 with positron emission tomography-computed tomography in four clinically normal dogs. Am J Vet Res 2012;73:1589–95.
17. Li Y, Schiepers C, Lake R, et al. Clincal utility of 18F-fluoride PET/CT in benign and malignant bone diseases. Bone 2012;50:128–39.
18. Freesmeyer M, Stecker FF, Schierz J-H, et al. First experience with early dynamic 18F-NaF-PET/CT in patients with chronic osteomyelitis. Ann Nucl Med 2014. http://dx.doi.org/10.1007/s12149-014-0810-4. [Epub ahead of print].
19. Czernin J, Satyamurthy N, Schiepers C. Molecular mechanisms of bone 18F-NaF deposition. J Nucl Med 2010;51:1826–9.
20. Ovadia D, Metser U, Lievshitz G, et al. Back pain in adolescents: assessment with integrated 18F-fluoride positron emission tomography-computed tomography. J Pediatr Orthop 2007;27:90–3.
21. Drubach LA, Connolly SA, Palmer EL III. Skeletal scintigraphy with 18F-NaF PET for the evaluation of bone pain in children. AJR Am J Roentgenol 2011; 197:713–9.
22. Coady CM, Micheli LJ. Stress fractures in the pediatric athlete. Clin Sports Med 1997;16:225–38.
23. Zukotynski K, Curtis C, Grant FD, et al. The value of SPECT in the detection of stress injury to the pars interarticularis in patients with low back pain. J Orthop Surg Res 2010;5:13.

24. Connolly LP, Drubach LA, Connolly SA, et al. Young athletes with low back pain: skeletal scintigraphy of conditions other than pars interarticularis stress. Clin Nucl Med 2004;29:689–93.

25. Connolly LP, d'Hemecourt PA, Connolly SA, et al. Skeletal scintigraphy of young patients with low-back pain and a lumbosacral transitional vertebra. J Nucl Med 2003;44:909–14.

26. Quon A, Dodd R, Iagaru A, et al. Initial investigation of 18F-NaF PET/CT for identification of vertebral sites amenable to surgical revision after spinal fusion surgery. Eur J Nucl Med Mol Imaging 2012; 39:1737–44.

27. Even-Sapir E, Mishani E, Flusser G, et al. 18F-fluoride positron emission tomography and positron emission tomography/computed tomography. Semin Nucl Med 2007;37:462–9.

28. Messa C, Goodman WG, Hoh CK, et al. Bone metabolic activity measured with positron emission tomography and [18F]fluoride ion in renal osteodystrophy: correlation with bone histomorhometry. J Clin Endocrinol Metab 1993;77:949–55.

29. Piert M, Zittel TT, Becker GA, et al. Assessment of porcine bone metabolism by dynamic 18F-fluoride ion PET: correlation with bone histomorphometry. J Nucl Med 2001;42:1091–100.

30. Installe J, Nzeusseu A, Bol A, et al. 18F-fluoride PET for monitoring therapeutic response in Paget's disease of bone. J Nucl Med 2005;46:1650–8.

31. Blake GM, Park-Holohan SJ, Fogelman I. Quantitative studies of bone in postmenopausal women using 18F-fluoride and 99mTc-methylene diphosphonate. J Nucl Med 2002;43:338–45.

32. DiVasta A, Feldman H, Blank B, et al. Through thick and thin: PET changes in bone turnover during starvation and refeeding. J Nucl Med 2013;54:S530.

33. Brenner W, Vernon C, Muzi M, et al. Comparison of different quantitative approaches to 18F-fluoride PET scans. J Nucl Med 2004;45:1493–500.

34. Forrest N, Welch A, Murray AD, et al. Femoral head viability after Birmingham resurfacing hip arthroplasty: assessment with use of [18F]fluoride positron emission tomography. J Bone Joint Surg Am 2006;88:S84–9.

35. Piert M, Winter E, Becker GA, et al. Allogenic bone graft viability after hip revision arthoplasty assessed by dynamic [18F]fluoride ion positron emission tomography. Eur J Nucl Med 1999;26:615–24.

36. Ullmark G, Sőrensen J, Lĭngstrőm B, et al. Bone regeneration 6 years after impaction bone grafting: a PET analysis. Acta Orthop 2007;78:201–5.

37. Schieppers C, Broos P, Miserez M, et al. Measurement of skeletal flow with positron emission tomography and 18F-fluoride in femoral head osteonecrosis. Arch Orthop Trauma Surg 1998;118:131–5.

38. Dasa V, Adbel-Nabi H, Anders MJ, et al. F-18 fluoride positron emission tomography of the hip for osteonecrosis. Clin Orthop Relat Res 2008;466: 1081–6.

39. Kleinman PL, Kleinman PK, Savageau JA. Suspected infant abuse: radiographic skeletal survey practices in pediatric health care facilities. Radiology 2004;233:477–85.

40. Drubach LA, Johnston PR, Newton AW, et al. Skeletal trauma in child abuse: detection with 18F-NaF PET. Radiology 2010;255:173–81.

41. Franzius C, Sciuk J, Daldrup-Link HE, et al. FDG-PET for detection of osseous metastases from malignant primary bone tumors: comparison with bone scintigraphy. Eur J Nucl Med 2000;8:1305–11.

Fluorocholine PET/Computed Tomography
Physiologic Uptake, Benign Findings, and Pitfalls

Mohsen Beheshti, MD, FASNC, FEBNM[a],*,
Athar Haroon, FRCR[b],
Jamshed B. Bomanji, MD, MBBS, PhD, FRCR, FRCP[b],
Werner Langsteger, MD[a]

KEYWORDS

• Choline • PET/CT • Physiologic variation • Benign findings • Pitfalls

KEY POINTS

- Radiolabeled choline uptake in PET/computed tomography studies is a marker of cell proliferation, as malignancies are commonly characterized by increased proliferative activity.
- The uptake of ^{18}F-choline can be seen in inflammatory conditions, possibly because of the proliferation of some cellular types involved in the genesis of phlogosis.
- The salivary glands, liver, adrenals, gastrointestinal tract, and urinary tract are the most common sites of physiologic choline uptake.
- Hormone therapy in patients with prostate cancer may cause increased reactive bone marrow uptake, which should be considered in the interpretation.

INTRODUCTION

There are 3 commonly used choline-based tracers: ^{11}C-choline, ^{18}F-methylcholine, and ^{18}F-ethylcholine.

- ^{11}C-Choline: lower urinary excretion, half-life 20 minutes
- ^{18}F-Methylcholine and ^{18}F-ethylcholine: higher urinary excretion, half-life 110 minutes

The uptake and phosphorylation of ^{18}F-labeled methylcholine (FCH) is similar to that of ^{11}C-labeled choline and superior to that of other choline analogues.[1] It has been suggested that ^{18}F-labeled choline may be superior to ^{11}C-choline PET in terms of sharpness of image.[2] Moreover, ^{11}C-choline studies are restricted to centers with an on-site cyclotron, whereas ^{18}F-labeled choline can be delivered to sites without a cyclotron unit. Each thus has advantages and disadvantages.

Choline PET in combination with computed tomography (PET/CT) is well established, and there is a wealth of literature available emphasizing the importance of choline in various malignancies. The ability to evaluate cell membrane turnover status is the main advantage of imaging with choline, and is a limitation of cross-sectional imaging (magnetic resonance [MR] imaging and CT). On the other hand, imaging with choline has the disadvantage of reduced spatial resolution in comparison with cross-sectional imaging. Thus the weakness of one is the strength of the other, and hybrid imaging in the form of PET/CT and PET/MR complements the role of choline. This

Conflict of Interest: The investigators declare no conflict of interest.
^a PET-CT Center LINZ, Department of Nuclear Medicine and Endocrinology, St. Vincent's Hospital, Seilerstaette 4, Linz A-4020, Austria; ^b T5 University College London Hospital, London, UK
* Corresponding author. Institute of Nuclear Medicine, T5 University College Hospital, 235 Euston Road, London NW1 2BU.
E-mail address: mohsen.beheshti@bhs.at

PET Clin 9 (2014) 299–306
http://dx.doi.org/10.1016/j.cpet.2014.03.001
1556-8598/14/$ – see front matter © 2014 Elsevier Inc. All rights reserved.

complementary role is very important in the head, neck, and pelvis, where precise anatomic detail is of utmost importance.

It is important that, considering the pharmacologic features and properties of choline, the uptake of the tracer can be seen in physiologic or benign conditions that integrate cell-membrane synthesis.

The pitfalls and artifacts of ^{18}F-FCH PET/CT have been previously described.[3] Knowledge of physiologic distribution (**Fig. 1**), benign findings, and the potentially false-positive uptake areas is of great importance for accurate interpretation of the images. This article discusses such findings and abnormal sites of ^{18}F-FCH uptake during PET/CT examinations, with the aim of expanding the knowledge about physiologic uptake of this radiotracer and depiction of those regions that occasionally may present increased activity unrelated to malignant tissue.

CENTRAL NERVOUS SYSTEM/HEAD AND NECK

Brain uptake of choline is low compared with uptake in the extracerebral tissues. There are 2 kinds of energy-dependent transport systems for choline incorporation in the cell membrane[4]:

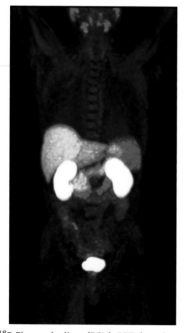

Fig. 1. ^{18}F-Fluorocholine (FCH) PET (maximum-intensity projection [MIP]). Physiologic pattern of tracer uptake with symmetric increased tracer uptake in the salivary glands; increased tracer uptake in the liver, spleen, pancreas, kidneys, urinary bladder, and gastrointestinal tract.

1. Phosphorylcholine synthesis: this is present on all mammalian cells.
2. Acetylcholine synthesis: this is present in the synaptosomes (cholinergic nerve endings) and the transport of choline is coupled to acetyl choline synthesis.

Because there is an increase in phosphorylcholine synthesis in tumors, clinical application of the choline-based tracers in the imaging of brain cancer is possible. In a study evaluating the physiologic uptake of ^{18}F-methylcholine,[5] a range of uptake was found in different head and neck tissues; for example, low-grade uptake in the normal brain parenchyma, and moderate uptake in the choroid plexus, cavernous sinus, extraocular eye muscles, masticatory muscles, and bone marrow. Uptake in the pituitary gland was generally moderately intense, whereas uptake in the lacrimal glands and the mucosa of the nasal cavity was found to be variable. Parotid glands demonstrated high-grade uptake. Tumors such as glioblastomas and meningiomas were found to be moderately intense, whereas uptake in grade II and III gliomas was globally faint.

Calabria and colleagues[6] reported abnormal tracer uptake in the area of mucosal thickening of the right maxillary sinus (maximum standardized uptake value [SUV_{max}] = 4). The clinical and imaging follow-up studies were then suggestive of sinusitis.

Asymmetric increased FCH uptake may also be seen in the submandibular glands, which is most likely functional and caused by unilateral glandular hypoplasia and/or aplasia (**Fig. 2**).

Thyroid gland shows mildly increased uptake on FCH PET. However, it is not clear whether there is any relationship between choline uptake in varying disease states, for example an inflammatory process such as autoimmune thyropathy, or if this is merely a physiologic pattern. Schillaci and colleagues[3] have reported a case of focal uptake in the thyroid gland that was found to be thyroiditis on ultrasonographic and biochemical tests (**Fig. 3**).

The authors currently are investigating the value of FCH PET/CT in the detection of parathyroid adenoma in patients with clinical evidence of primary hyperparathyroidism and negative or equivocal ^{99m}Tc-methoxyisobutylisonitrile (MIBI) scintigraphy. The early results are promising, and FCH PET/CT seems to be superior to ^{99}Tc-MIBI scintigraphy even with single-photon emission CT/CT.

The uptake of ^{18}F-choline in inflammatory conditions that could be due to the proliferation of some cellular types involved in the genesis of phlogosis, such as the white cell series, has already been described.[6,7] Choline PET can be positive in

Diffuse increased uptake of choline in the lungs reflects a generalized problem related to lung parenchyma (**Fig. 5**). The surface tension of lung parenchyma is maintained by surfactant, which is secreted by type II alveolar cells. Increased concentration of surfactant is seen in the alveoli in cases of pulmonary edema. Diffuse increased uptake of choline in patients with heart failure with congestive changes in the lungs is a sequela of pulmonary venous imbalance.

A complete cholinergic autocrine loop has been identified in small cell lung cancer and mesothelioma cells.[8] The clinical role of choline has been evaluated for malignancies such as adenocarcinoma and bronchioloalveolar cell carcinoma.[9,10] The uptake of choline in thoracic malignancies is not tumor specific. In one study, ^{11}C-choline PET/CT was not significantly better at diagnosing pulmonary lesions than enhanced CT; however, ^{11}C-choline PET/CT had improved sensitivity, specificity, accuracy, positive predictive value, and negative predictive value relative to enhanced CT in the evaluation of locoregional lymph nodes.[11] In another study comparing ^{11}C-choline with ^{18}F-fluorodeoxyglucose (FDG), there was no significant difference in the detection of primary lung cancer; however ^{18}F-FDG was found to be superior to ^{11}C-choline in the detection of nodal involvement.[12]

Mediastinal, hilar, and axillary lymph nodes may show mild increased tracer uptakes, which are mostly reactive or related to an inflammatory process. The mean registered SUV_{max} of such lymph nodes is approximately 2.8.[6]

Based on the authors' experience, tracer intensity in the reactive lymph nodes is usually higher than blood pool activity and similar to the bone marrow uptake in the thoracic spine, with ±20% difference. Inflammatory lymph nodes resulting from granulomatous disease may show intensive tracer uptake. However, they mostly show the typical symmetric pattern of tracer uptake in the mediastinum and hilum (**Fig. 6**). Moreover, no significant myocardial uptake was seen in choline PET studies.

Mild increased tracer uptake may be seen on the brachial and or cephalic vein at the injection side, which may be related to rapid and unspecific endothelial uptake (see **Fig. 3**).

Thymoma may also show an intensive choline uptake with a SUV_{max} of approximately 8.[6] Pleuritis and esophagitis are other causes of increased choline uptake.[3]

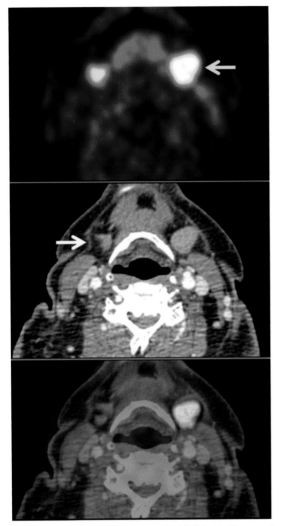

Fig. 2. FCH PET/CT. (*Top*) PET, (*middle*) CT, (*bottom*) fusion PET/CT. Asymmetric increased tracer uptake in the left submandibular gland (*top, arrow*) owing to right-side atrophy (*middle, arrow*).

inflammatory conditions, and is one of the reasons for a false-positive result in, for example, sinusitis, thyroiditis (see **Fig. 3**), and otomastoiditis.[3] These findings should be correlated clinically with biochemical results and relevant histology if available. Recent trauma and bone fracture also show increased choline uptake (**Fig. 4**).

THORAX

Lung parenchyma is nonavid on all 3 tracers, apart from the lung bases where curvilinear uptake is seen along the thoracic wall, predominantly at the lung bases and on the periphery. This finding may represent dependent change, as the patients are normally scanned in the supine position.

ABDOMEN

The angiotensin-converting enzyme converts acetylcholine to the inactive metabolites choline

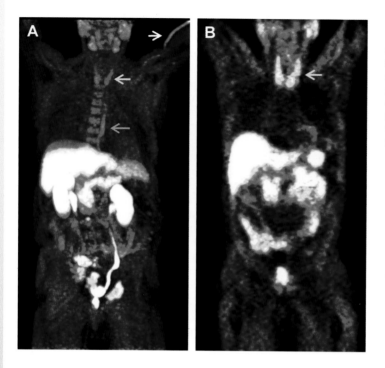

Fig. 3. FCH PET (MIP). (*A*) Mild increased tracer uptake along with cephalic vein at the injection side, unspecific (*white arrow*); in the thyroid gland, suggesting autoimmune thyropathy (*yellow arrow*); and in the esophagus, suggesting esophagitis (*blue arrow*). (*B*) Intensive tracer uptake on the thyroid, suggesting thyroiditis (*arrow*).

and acetate in an intracellular and extracellular manner. These cholinergic components are expressed in noncancerous liver cells,[8] so the physiologic pattern of choline uptake is that of diffuse increased uptake throughout the liver parenchyma (**Fig. 7**). Just as for FDG, there is mild increased uptake at the periphery of the liver in comparison with the lobes toward the porta hepatis, which may be due to perfusion-related parameters rather than a true reflection of difference in cell membrane phospholipid contents.

Choline-containing compounds have been detected in liver tumors such as hepatoma by ^{1}H MR spectroscopy.[13,14] Target-to-noise ratio plays an important role in the detection of clinically significant lesions, which can be either avid or photopenic. For avid lesions no significant difference was found between the 2 choline tracers ^{18}F-ethylcholine and ^{11}C-choline in the detection of hepatocellular carcinoma.[15] ^{18}F-Choline has been found to have a better detection rate and similar prognostic value in comparison with FDG.[16] In unifocal hepatocellular carcinoma (HCC), a photopenic pattern of ^{18}F-choline was found to be associated with microvascular invasion, and predicted early HCC recurrence after surgical resection as accurately as did FDG uptake.[16] The imaging reporter should be aware of this variation. Clinical correlation and reference to previous cross-sectional imaging is suggested for characterization of indeterminate lesions.

The gastrointestinal tract demonstrates a variable pattern of uptake. Once the choline is injected intravenously there is hepatic and biliary uptake, with subsequent excretion into the small bowel. The mid/distal part of the small bowel, cecum, ascending colon, and middle part of the transverse colon are nonavid. The zone of transition of metabolic activity varies slightly between the 3 tracers, but there is clearly a transition from nonavid bowel to heterogeneously avid bowel at approximately the mid-transverse colon. Physiologic uptake in the colon, for which rapid turnover of the epithelial cells may be a contributory factor, has been demonstrated to be lower than that in small intestine; this is in contrast to FDG uptake, which is higher in the small and large intestine.[17]

The pancreas is one of the most avid structures seen on choline PET as evaluated by Schillaci and colleagues.[3] The pancreatic body and tail show variably moderate to intense uptake while the pancreatic head is intensely avid. Atrophic changes in the pancreas cause replacement of the pancreatic parenchyma with fat.[18] These changes can cause focal or diffuse reduction in choline uptake. Reduced uptake in the pancreas may be due to a physiologic process.

There is uptake of moderate intensity in the spleen. The adrenal glands are usually nonavid with all choline-based tracers; however, mild increased choline uptake can be seen unilaterally and/or bilaterally in the adrenal glands, with a mean SUV_{max} of

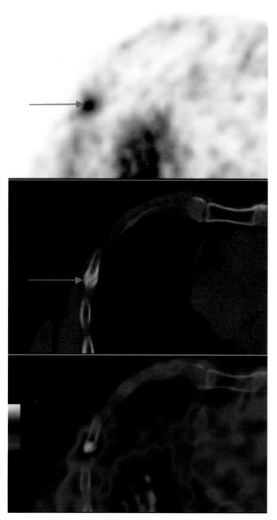

2.8 or less.[6] Adrenal adenoma may also show mild to moderate increased choline uptake correlated with corresponding findings on CT.

PELVIS (INCLUDING THE GENITOURINARY SYSTEM)

Kidneys demonstrate excreted activity, which enters the ureters and bladder. Some centers prefer to use hydration (500 mL normal saline 0.9% intravenously) before scanning to minimize urinary pooling in the kidneys.[3] Physiologic bladder activity poses a challenge, and different centers adopt varying protocols to counter this problem; for example, initial dynamic imaging of the pelvis before excreted activity is seen in the bladder, followed by delayed imaging of the whole body. The patients are asked to empty their bladder before delayed imaging to minimize the residual excreted activity in the urinary bladder. The bulbourethral gland may also show focal increased tracer uptake, especially in the early dynamic images.

The normal prostate may show only faint increased uptake. Prostate cancer demonstrates an area of focal or diffuse increased tracer uptake. Local inflammation of the prostate can also cause increased accumulation of focal tracer, and is the most common cause of false-positive choline uptake (**Fig. 8**). The role of choline in prostate cancer is well established,[19–21] and the main indications for the use of choline is staging in high-risk patients, relapse of prostate cancer, rising prostate-specific antigen levels, and negative conventional imaging.[21]

Inguinal lymph nodes showing mild to moderate increased choline uptake, usually with rapid washout, are usually considered to be reactive (see **Fig. 8**).

Fig. 4. FCH PET/CT. (*Top*) PET, (*middle*) CT, (*bottom*) fusion PET/CT. Focal increased tracer uptake on a rib (*top, arrow*) correlated with a recent fracture on CT (*middle, arrow*).

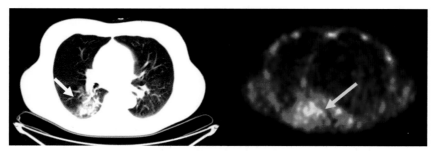

Fig. 5. FCH PET/CT. (*Left*) PET, (*right*) CT. Diffuse increased tracer uptake on the lower lobe of the right lung (*yellow arrow*) correlated with inflammatory changes on CT (*white arrow*), suggesting pneumonitis.

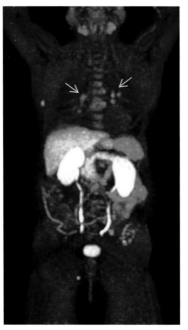

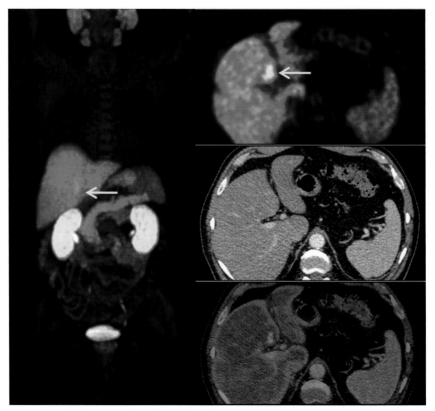

EFFECT OF DRUGS

Roef and colleagues[22] have reported an interesting case in a patient on colchicine undergoing ^{18}F-methylcholine PET, who had blood pool activity only on colchicine. The activity was normalized to physiologic when the colchicine was stopped and the scan was repeated. The investigators suggested that colchicine impairs the normal choline pathway, and must be stopped before ^{18}F-methylcholine PET/CT imaging takes place. Drugs with a possible similar effect include docetaxel and paclitaxel.[22] Recent literature has also demonstrated a promising role of choline PET in patients with prostate cancer with biochemical recurrence. The investigators reported that mean SUV_{max} was slightly higher in patients with ongoing hormone therapy (HT) in comparison with patients without HT (9.3 ± 5.7 vs 7.8 ± 4.7, $P = .08$). In addition, there was no significant correlation between the duration of HT and the time interval between HT withdrawal and FCH PET/CT positivity.[20]

Fig. 6. FCH PET (MIP). Focal increased tracer uptake on both sides of mediastinum and hilum (*arrows*), suggesting granulomatous disease.

Fig. 7. FCH PET/CT. (*Left*) MIP. (*Right*) PET (*top*), CT (*middle*), fusion PET/CT (*bottom*). Increased tracer uptake in the periphery of the liver (*arrow*) without any morphologic correlation on CT and follow-up magnetic resonance imaging, most likely related to liver perfusion.

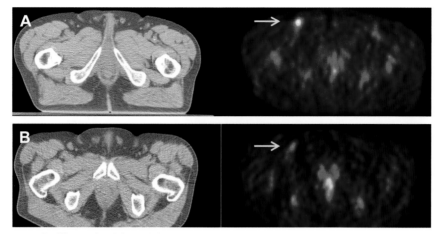

Fig. 8. FCH PET/CT. (*Left*) PET, (*right*) CT. (*A*) Focal increased tracer uptake in the right inguinal region 1 minute after injection (*arrow*, standardized uptake value [SUV] = 4.4). (*B*) Delayed image (120 minutes postinjection) shows marked washout with SUV = 2.4 (*arrow*), suggesting a reactive lymph node.

Moreover, patients with ongoing HT may show mildly increased and nonhomogeneous bone marrow uptake in the axial skeleton, which may cause false-positive results (**Fig. 9**). Based on their experience, the authors suggest that performing an additional delayed acquisition from the suspicious regions is useful in differentiating malignant from reactive bony lesions.

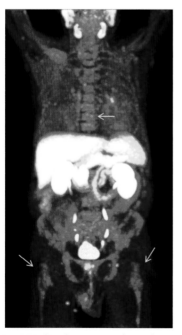

Fig. 9. FCH PET (MIP). Increased nonhomogeneous bone marrow uptake in the axial skeleton and lower extremities (*arrows*), made reactive by ongoing hormone therapy.

SUMMARY

Choline PET has a role in the diagnosis of malignancies. Knowledge of normal biodistribution plays a vital role in disease characterization and in differentiating normal variants from disease processes. CT and MR scans provide complementary information, and choline-positive sites should be correlated clinically to exclude inflammatory disorders.

REFERENCES

1. DeGrado TR, Baldwin SW, Wang S, et al. Synthesis and evaluation of (18)F-labeled choline analogs as oncologic PET tracers. J Nucl Med 2001;42(12): 1805–14.
2. Hara T, Kosaka N, Kishi H. Development of (18)F-fluoroethylcholine for cancer imaging with PET: synthesis, biochemistry, and prostate cancer imaging. J Nucl Med 2002;43(2):187–99.
3. Schillaci O, Calabria F, Tavolozza M, et al. ^{18}F-choline PET/CT physiological distribution and pitfalls in image interpretation: experience in 80 patients with prostate cancer. Nucl Med Commun 2010;31(1):39–45.
4. Friedland RP, Mathis CA, Budinger TF, et al. Labeled choline and phosphorylcholine: body distribution and brain autoradiography: concise communication. J Nucl Med 1983;24(9):812–5.
5. Mertens K, Ham H, Deblaere K, et al. Distribution patterns of ^{18}F-labelled fluoromethylcholine in normal structures and tumors of the head: a PET/MRI evaluation. Clin Nucl Med 2012;37(8):e196–203.
6. Calabria F, Chiaravalloti A, Schillaci O. (18)F-choline PET/CT pitfalls in image interpretation: an update on 300 examined patients with prostate cancer. Clin Nucl Med 2014;39(2):122–30.

7. Wyss MT, Weber B, Honer M, et al. ^{18}F-choline in experimental soft tissue infection assessed with autoradiography and high-resolution PET. Eur J Nucl Med Mol Imaging 2004;31(3):312–6.

8. Gu J. Primary liver cancer: challenges and perspectives. Hangzhou: Zhejiang University Press and Heidelberg: Springer; 2012.

9. Balogova S, Huchet V, Kerrou K, et al. Detection of bronchioloalveolar cancer by means of PET/CT and ^{18}F-fluorocholine, and comparison with ^{18}F-fluorodeoxyglucose. Nucl Med Commun 2010;31(5):389–97.

10. Wang T, Li J, Chen F, et al. Choline transporters in human lung adenocarcinoma: expression and functional implications. Acta Biochim Biophys Sin (Shanghai) 2007;39(9):668–74.

11. Peng Z, Liu Q, Li M, et al. Comparison of (11)C-choline PET/CT and enhanced CT in the evaluation of patients with pulmonary abnormalities and locoregional lymph node involvement in lung cancer. Clin Lung Cancer 2012;13(4):312–20.

12. Pieterman RM, Que TH, Elsinga PH, et al. Comparison of (11)C-choline and (18)F-FDG PET in primary diagnosis and staging of patients with thoracic cancer. J Nucl Med 2002;43(2):167–72.

13. de Certaines JD, Larsen VA, Podo F, et al. In vivo ^{31}P MRS of experimental tumours. NMR Biomed 1993; 6(6):345–65.

14. Sutinen E, Nurmi M, Roivainen A, et al. Kinetics of [(11)C]choline uptake in prostate cancer: a PET study. Eur J Nucl Med Mol Imaging 2004;31(3):317–24.

15. Kolthammer JA, Corn DJ, Tenley N, et al. PET imaging of hepatocellular carcinoma with ^{18}F-fluoroethylcholine and ^{11}C-choline. Eur J Nucl Med Mol Imaging 2011;38(7):1248–56.

16. Fartoux L, Balogova S, Nataf V, et al. A pilot comparison of ^{18}F-fluorodeoxyglucose and ^{18}F-fluorocholine PET/CT to predict early recurrence of unifocal hepatocellular carcinoma after surgical resection. Nucl Med Commun 2012;33(7):757–65.

17. Terauchi T, Tateishi U, Maeda T, et al. A case of colon cancer detected by carbon-11 choline positron emission tomography/computed tomography: an initial report. Jpn J Clin Oncol 2007;37(10):797–800.

18. Katz DS, Hines J, Math KR, et al. Using CT to reveal fat-containing abnormalities of the pancreas. AJR Am J Roentgenol 1999;172(2):393–6.

19. Beheshti M, Haim S, Zakavi R, et al. Impact of ^{18}F-choline PET/CT in prostate cancer patients with biochemical recurrence: influence of androgen deprivation therapy and correlation with PSA kinetics. J Nucl Med 2013;54(6):833–40.

20. Beheshti M, Imamovic L, Broinger G, et al. [18]F choline PET/CT in the preoperative staging of prostate cancer in patients with intermediate or high risk of extracapsular disease: a prospective study of 130 patients. Radiology 2010;254(3):925–33.

21. Ceci F, Castellucci P, Mamede M, et al. (11)C-Choline PET/CT in patients with hormone-resistant prostate cancer showing biochemical relapse after radical prostatectomy. Eur J Nucl Med Mol Imaging 2013;40(2):149–55.

22. Roef MJ, van der Poel H, van der Laken CJ, et al. Colchicine must be stopped before imaging with [^{18}F]-methylcholine PET/CT. Nucl Med Commun 2010;31(12):1075–7.

^{18}F-DOPA PET/Computed Tomography Imaging

Sotirios Chondrogiannis, MD, Maria Cristina Marzola, MD, Domenico Rubello, MD*

KEYWORDS

- Biodistribution • L-6-Fluoro-3,4-dihydroxyphenylalanine PET/CT • ^{18}F-DOPA • Physiologic pattern
- ^{18}F-DOPA pitfalls • ^{18}F-DOPA variants

KEY POINTS

- ^{18}F-DOPA is a promising radiopharmaceutical for the evaluation of neuroendocrine tumors, brain tumors, pancreatic cell hyperplasia, and the integrity of the striatal dopaminergic system.
- ^{18}F-DOPA traces a very specific metabolic pathway with minimal uptake in normal tissues, and therefore provides good lesion-to-background ratios.
- The biodistribution pattern is very distinct, and variations depend mainly on the variable excretion of the tracer through the biliary or the urinary tract.
- As for any radiopharmaceutical, thorough knowledge of the biodistribution, variants, or possible pitfalls helps avoid misinterpretations.

INTRODUCTION

The increasing availability of numerous positron-emitting radiopharmaceuticals, especially ^{18}F-fluorodeoxyglucose (^{18}F-FDG), and the new generation of hybrid PET/computed tomography (CT) systems have considerably improved the management of a wide range of oncologic and nononcologic disorders. The documented limitations of ^{18}F-FDG, the main PET radiopharmaceutical, such as its inability to detect well-differentiated tumors such as neuroendocrine tumors, to differentiate inflammation from neoplasms, to reveal lesions in organs with high physiologic uptake such as brain tumors, or to assess more specific metabolic processes other than glycolytic metabolism, have intensified the search for new, more specific radiopharmaceuticals.[1] One of these new, promising radiotracers is the amino acid–based radiopharmaceutical ^{18}F-DOPA (L-6-[^{18}F]fluoro-3,4-dihydroxyphenylalanine), which was originally used in patients with Parkinson disease to assess the integrity of the striatal dopaminergic system. In recent years, especially after the introduction of the hybrid PET/CT scanners, it has also adopted an important role in the management of neuroendocrine tumors, brain tumors, and pancreatic cell hyperplasia.[2–5]

However, despite the sound pathophysiologic rational basis and the promising diagnostic results of ^{18}F-DOPA PET, there still remains a relative paucity of data because of the rarity of these disorders, the existence of other PET/single PET radiopharmaceuticals, and the complicated manufacture of ^{18}F-DOPA.[6,7]

The purpose of this article is to present the main clinical applications of ^{18}F-DOPA PET/CT, focusing on the physiologic biodistribution of the tracer and its normal variants, and to describe possible pitfalls that could lead to misinterpretations of the scans in the various clinical settings.

THE RADIOPHARMACEUTICAL

Dihydroxyphenylalanine (DOPA) is an amino acid containing 2 hydroxyl groups on the 3- and 4-positions of the phenol ring, which can be labeled with

There are no conflicts of interest.
Department of Nuclear Medicine, PET/CT Centre, Santa Maria della Misericordia Hospital, Viale Tre Martiri 140, Rovigo 45100, Italy
* Corresponding author.
E-mail address: domenico.rubello@libero.it

PET Clin 9 (2014) 307–321
http://dx.doi.org/10.1016/j.cpet.2014.03.007
1556-8598/14/$ – see front matter © 2014 Elsevier Inc. All rights reserved.

the positron-emitter isotope fluorine-18 (^{18}F) in the sixth position forming ^{18}F-DOPA, which allows PET imaging.[8]

L-DOPA (L-3,4-dihydroxyphenylalanine) is the precursor of the neurotransmitters dopamine, norepinephrine (adrenaline), and norepinephrine (noradrenaline), collectively known as catecholamines. ^{18}F-DOPA is a large neutral amino acid that resembles natural L-dopa biochemically and presents similar kinetics. It enters the catecholamine metabolic pathway of endogenous L-DOPA both in the brain and peripherally.[9,10] The relatively long half-life (110 minutes) of ^{18}F-DOPA makes it suitable for transportation even in centers with no cyclotron facility on site, allows more flexible imaging timings, and offers the possibility for late images, which are very important in some cases.

MAIN CLINICAL APPLICATIONS OF ^{18}F-DOPA PET/CT
Imaging the Striatum

Since the 1980s ^{18}F-DOPA has been synthesized and used as positron-emitting tracer for PET imaging examination of patients affected by Parkinson disease.[11] The rationale of ^{18}F-DOPA PET is based on the utilization of ^{18}F-DOPA (a positron emitter) by the brain as a precursor for dopamine. In the brain, L-DOPA is capable of crossing the blood-brain barrier, owing to the large neutral amino acid transport system.[9,12,13] After entering the cells, the aromatic amino acid decarboxylase enzyme (AADC) transforms L-DOPA into dopamine, which is stored in presynaptic vesicles through the vesicular monoamine transporter and is eventually released into the extracellular space of the synapse during neurotransmission.[13,14] Therefore, ^{18}F-DOPA can be clinically used to trace the dopaminergic pathway and evaluate striatal dopaminergic presynaptic function.[14–17]

Imaging Brain Tumors

The first visualization of a brain tumor with ^{18}F-DOPA PET was an incidental finding in a patient evaluated for movement disorders.[18,19] Amino acid PET tracers and amino acid analogue PET tracers are particularly attractive for imaging brain tumors because of the high uptake in tumor and the low or absent uptake in normal brain tissue and, thus, higher contrast in tumor relative to normal tissue.[3,20,21] The uptake mechanism is based on the observation that amino acid transport is generally highly expressed in malignant tissues, causing an increased uptake of amino acids in brain tumors in comparison with that in normal brain.[3,21–24] ^{18}F-DOPA PET in brain tumors

demonstrated promising results evaluating high-grade and low-grade tumors and recurrent tumors, in addition to differentiating between recurrence and radiation necrosis.[3,18,25,26]

Imaging Neuroendrocrine Tumors

Neuroendocrine tumors (NETs) are a rare and heterogeneous group of neoplasms with various clinical presentations and growth rates that can arise throughout the body. NETs are located mainly in the gastroenteropancreatic tract but can also be found in other organs, such as the bronchopulmonary system (carcinoids, microcytoma), the medulla of the adrenal (pheochromocytoma), the extra-adrenal paraganglia (paragangliomas, carotid glomus tumors), the head and neck region (medullary thyroid carcinoma, paragangliomas), and the neural crest of the sympathetic nervous system (neuroblastoma).

The rational basis that leads to the uptake of ^{18}F-DOPA by NETs is their ability to accumulate amino acids (amine precursors) such as L-DOPA and transform them into biogenic amines (such as catecholamine and serotonin) after decarboxylation by means of the aromatic L-amino acid decarboxylase (AADC) enzyme.[27,28] Neuroendocrine tumors show an overexpression of the AADC enzyme and a strong upregulation of amino acid transporters to handle the increased demand of biogenic amine precursors in their overactive metabolic pathways.[8] Because surgery is the only curative approach for NETs, early detection and accurate staging of the disease are fundamental in establishing the treatment option. Moreover, PET/CT offers whole-body evaluation, combining functional information and corresponding anatomic localization, thus providing a diagnostic tool that has the potential to become a stand-alone method for the complete assessment of NETs. The main NETs studied with ^{18}F-DOPA are carcinoids, pheochromocytomas, paragangliomas, and medullary thyroid carcinomas (MTCs). Carcinoid tumors are relatively indolent tumors arising from neuroendocrine cells.[29] Paragangliomas are rare neuroendocrine tumors arising from chromaffin cells of the sympathetic and parasympathetic paraganglia, located from the base of the skull to the urinary bladder. Catecholamine-secreting paragangliomas arising from the chromaffin cells of the adrenal medulla are referred to as pheochromocytomas, whereas sympathetic paragangliomas arising outside the adrenals are referred to as extra-adrenal paragangliomas.[30,31] An MTC is a slow-growing neuroendocrine tumor that arises from parafollicular C cells in the thyroid and may be either sporadic

(75%) or familiar (25%), and associated with multiple endocrine neoplasia (MEN2). After thyroidectomy, the main treatment option for MTC, levels of calcitonin and carcinoembryonic antigen may increase, indicating recurrent disease. The early detection of recurrence represents an important step in the management and outcome of patients with MTC.[32,33]

Imaging (Congenital) Hyperinsulinemic Hypoglycemia

Hyperinsulinemic hypoglycemia is another disorder for which ^{18}F-DOPA that has shown promising results. This condition can be caused in adults by a solitary insulinoma (neuroendocrine tumor) or B-cell hyperplasia,[34] and in infants by focal or diffuse B-cell hyperplasia. As part of the amine precursor uptake and decarboxylation system, normal islets in the pancreas also take up amine precursors (such as ^{18}F-DOPA) and decarboxylate them to amines by means of AADC.[4] In hyperfunctioning islets (as in cases of insulinomas or primary hyperinsulinemia), the uptake can be pronounced, and ^{18}F-DOPA PET can be of value for evaluating such patients.[35] It is still an open question in the literature whether ^{18}F-DOPA can be of any use in evaluating adult patients with hyperinsulinemic hypoglycemia, because the diffuse physiologic uptake in the pancreas can mask pathologic lesions.[4,34] On the other hand, ^{18}F-DOPA PET has an important role in the evaluation of congenital hyperinsulinism, because the discrimination between focal or diffuse hyperplasia and the precise preoperative localization of the focal hyperplasia can guide and facilitate the surgical approach.[4,34,36]

^{18}F-DOPA PET/CT ACQUISITION PROTOCOL
Carbidopa Pretreatment

Carbidopa (L-α-hydrazino-α-methyl-β-(3,4-dihydroxyphenyl) propionic acid) is a known inhibitor of AADC that inhibits the conversion of L-DOPA to dopamine in extracerebral tissues.[37,38] Carbidopa pretreatment improves imaging of the striatum by preventing early decarboxylation of ^{18}F-DOPA to ^{18}F-dopamine outside the brain, thereby increasing striatal uptake by increasing the concentration of ^{18}F-DOPA in plasma and decreasing renal excretion.[39] Carbidopa is also used to increase ^{18}F-DOPA uptake by tumor cells in the imaging of NETs.[29,39,40] Carbidopa premedication often consists of an oral administration of 100 to 250 mg of carbidopa 1 hour before acquisition.

Premedication with carbidopa improves the sensitivity of ^{18}F-DOPA PET for the localization of paraganglioma, because it enhances the uptake and allows better discrimination between paraganglioma and physiologic tracer uptake by normal surrounding tissues.[40] A markedly increased uptake of ^{18}F-DOPA by the basal ganglia, lungs, myocardium, and liver after premedication with carbidopa has also been reported, whereas the pancreas usually cannot be discerned.[40] Physiologic excretion into bile ducts, the gallbladder, and the urogenital system continued to be seen after carbidopa.

Premedication with carbidopa in children seems to influence the biodistribution of ^{18}F-DOPA in the liver and pancreas in a manner similar to that reported in adults.[41] Carbidopa premedication is not recommended in the evaluation of pancreatic lesions such as insulinomas or B-cell hyperplasia, because the reduced uptake in the whole pancreas (both healthy and pathologic) might hide the pathologic areas, leading to false-negative results.[29,40]

Preparation

Most centers that perform ^{18}F-DOPA PET/CT ask patients to fast for 4 to 6 hours before receiving the intravenous injection of ^{18}F-DOPA. Medication that could interfere with the uptake of the tracer can be withdrawn for 24 hours, but for most indications no special interactions have been reported and no suspension of pharmaceuticals is needed. Some centers premedicate patients with carbidopa (usually 100–200 mg 1 hour before the injection). The only specific preparation described in the literature is for congenital hyperinsulinism for which, because it is a rare condition, investigators from several centers have proposed a standard protocol for ^{18}F-DOPA PET/CT that consists in discontinuing some medications for at least 2 days (diazoxide, octreotide, and glucagon), a fasting condition for at least 6 hours, and a glucose infusion to maintain euglycemia. In this case, the use of carbidopa in not recommended because it could block not only the physiologic pancreatic uptake but also uptake of the pathologic area within the pancreas.[42]

Dose and Timing

The activity administered varies largely in the literature. The authors administer a fixed dose of 185 MBq of ^{18}F-DOPA, and all acquisitions are performed at 1 hour after injection. The choice of a 1-hour time interval between injection and acquisition was made on the basis of a previous preclinical study performed by the authors on 15 macaque monkeys as part of the Xenome multicenter European Community Project. During that study it was observed that the steady state of the pharmaceutical on the striatum is reached

1 hour after injection.[43] The tracer should be injected slowly to avoid pharmacologic effects, which could provoke a carcinoid crisis, especially when specific activity is low.[44] Other activity doses and acquisition timings have been described: in patients with NETs, Kauhanen and colleagues[2] report average administered doses of 234 ± 56 MBq and acquisition at 1 hour postinjection. Schiesser and colleagues[45] used standard doses of 200 to 220 MBq and acquisition at 45 minutes. For recurrent MTC, variable mean doses (185–740 MBq), acquisition timing (50–90 minutes), and time per bed position (3–20 minutes) have been reported,[46] with and without carbidopa premedication.[47] The same variability was present in the studies included in a recent meta-analysis on paragangliomas: mean doses (180–470 MBq), acquisition timing (30–90 minutes), and carbidopa premedication.[31] The European Association of Nuclear Medicine guidelines on paraganglioma imaging recommend a dose of 4 MBq/kg and imaging 30 to 60 minutes after injection.[48] In the evaluation of brain tumors the best time interval for acquisition is between 10 and 30 minutes after injection, because tumor uptake is near maximum and occurs sufficiently early to avoid peak uptake in the striatum.[3]

Acquisition

Imaging of ^{18}F-DOPA is similar to that performed with most PET radiopharmaceuticals, namely from the base of the skull to mid-thighs. Early images centered over the abdomen may be acquired to overcome difficulties in localizing abdominal paragangliomas located near the hepatobiliary system because of physiologic tracer.[48] Early images centered over the neck may also be acquired in patients with MTC, because these tumors often show rapid washout and are better visualized on these early images.[49,50] Moreover, the long half-life of the tracer (110 minutes) allows late particular images that can be useful in case of interpretative doubts (eg, activity in the urinary system or the bowel).

In patients who are referred to the authors for MTC or in the presence/suspicion of head and neck localization of disease, an additional late acquisition of the head and neck region is routinely performed using a specific acquisition protocol that consists of a particular acquisition from the vertex to the upper lung, with the same whole-body scout and CT parameters but with different PET parameters: usually, 2 PET bed positions of 5 minutes each, matrix 256×256 (instead of 3.5 minutes per bed and 128×128 matrix of the whole-body acquisition). The bigger matrix and the longer PET acquisition protocol offer a better spatial resolution and a better identification of small pathologic deposits with faint uptake, such as small laterocervical lymph nodes.

NORMAL BIODISTRIBUTION OF WHOLE-BODY ^{18}F-DOPA PET/CT

In the last decade, some new radiotracers other than ^{18}F-FDG have been introduced to research and clinical practice. The knowledge of the physiologic uptake of a new radiopharmaceutical and its variants represents an important step toward the correct interpretation of pathologic findings. In 2011 the authors' group published a study on the physiologic biodistribution pattern and the physiologic variants of ^{18}F-DOPA PET/CT in a cohort of 107 patients (53 men and 54 women, mean age 54.6 years, range 9–85 years).[51] Patients were referred for suspected neuroendocrine tumors, mainly pheochromocytoma, paraganglioma, and MTC. PET scans were performed without premedication with carbidopa. A semiquantitative uptake analysis using the upper limit of the standardized uptake value (SUV_{max}) in the sites of physiologic uptake was performed in both ^{18}F-DOPA negative (n = 32) and positive (n = 75) patients using a planar circular region of interest of 1 cm diameter, automatically generated by the computer, positioned on the slice with the highest uptake of each organ.

In the head and neck region uptake was seen, as expected, only in the basal ganglia (mean SUV_{max} 2.77, range 1.5–3.6), and only mild, unspecific uptake was observed in the oral cavity.

Mild uptake was apparent in the thorax, myocardium, peripheral muscles, and esophagus; in some cases a very faint uptake was seen in the mammary glands.

In the abdomen and pelvis region all patients showed uptake in the liver (mean SUV_{max} 2.15, range 1.1–2.9) and the pancreas, mainly to the uncinate process (mean SUV_{max} 5.67, range 2.9–14.1), and less intensely in the body-tail region (mean SUV_{max} 4.07, range 2.1–6.2) and adrenal glands (mean SUV_{max} 1.92, range 0.7–4.3). Depending on individual elimination timing, very intense and variable uptake was seen in the excretory organs: gallbladder and biliary tract (mean SUV_{max} 8.5), kidneys (mean SUV_{max} 4.4), and ureters and urinary bladder (mean SUV_{max} 111). In this series, bowel uptake (mean SUV_{max} 2.3) was an unusual finding and, when seen, presented only mild diffuse uptake. Statistical analysis using the Mann-Whitney test showed that the physiologic DOPA biodistribution was not significantly different in the DOPA-positive and the DOPA-negative scans ($P > .05$). Mild uptake was also seen in the duodenum and the bowel. However, greater variability was observed in the pancreas, especially in the uncinate process and the adrenal glands. Regarding the adrenals, the data showed significant variability in DOPA uptake. Physiologic DOPA uptake was observed in 44% of negative patients with a relatively high SUV_{max} of up to 4.3. However, the morphologic imaging and metanephrine urinary level were normal in all these cases, thus excluding medullary adrenal disease. Nevertheless, this site of uptake must be taken into consideration. In the literature it is reported that children can present 18F-DOPA uptake in the growth plates (**Fig. 1**, **Tables 1** and **2**).[8]

EFFECT OF CARBIDOPA PREMEDICATION ON THE BIODISTRIBUTION OF 18F-DOPA

As already mentioned, premedication with carbidopa may largely improve the diagnostic performance of 18F-DOPA PET in the localization of paragangliomas and carcinoid tumors, and can enhance striatum uptake.[29,40] In fact, after carbidopa administration the uptake of 18F-DOPA by the basal ganglia, lungs, myocardium, and liver increased markedly, as indicated by significantly higher SUVs.[40] Without premedication with carbidopa the pancreas is clearly visible, with variable uptake on 18F-DOPA PET, whereas after carbidopa the pancreas in most the cases cannot be visualized.[40] Physiologic excretion into the ducts of the biliary tract, the gallbladder, and the urinary system continues to be seen after carbidopa, with no differences reported. Similar effects of carbidopa premedication are reported in children (**Fig. 2**, see **Tables 1** and **2**).[41]

Image Interpretation

18F-DOPA is difficult to synthesize but easy to "read" because it traces a very specific metabolic process and presents unspecific accumulation only to its excretory pathways. In normal tissues, 18F-DOPA has minimal uptake and therefore provides good lesion-to-background ratios. For the correct interpretation of the PET images it is mandatory, as for every radiopharmaceutical, to have a good knowledge of its uptake mechanisms, its biodistribution patterns and kinetics, and the factors that could affect them in different organs and abnormalities (as in case of carbidopa premedication). Moreover, patients who are referred for 18F-DOPA PET/CT have already a clinical suspicion of disease based on their clinical record, biochemical findings, or imaging procedures, and therefore present with a very precise clinical indication.

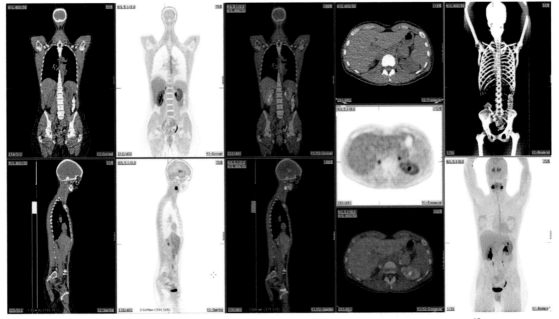

Fig. 1. A patient with a bilateral head/neck paraganglioma pretreated with carbidopa before 18F-DOPA PET/CT. Note the physiologic uptake in the striatum, oral cavity, esophagus, bowel, mammary glands, myocardium, liver, kidneys, both ureters, and bladder. No uptake is seen in the pancreas after carbidopa administration. Note the mild physiologic bilateral uptake in the adrenals (*fourth column* CT, PET, PET/CT). (*Courtesy of* Karel Pacak, MD, PhD, DSc, and Elise Blanchet, MD, Bethesda, MD.)

Table 1
Biodistribution of ^{18}F-DOPA in healthy humans

Normal Biodistribution	
Mild uptake	Myocardium, liver, bowel, adrenals (and less frequently the duodenum, mammary glands, oral cavity)
Moderate uptake	Striatum, pancreas (especially the uncinate process)
Intense uptake	Gallbladder and biliary tract, urinary tract

After premedication with carbidopa there is usually absence of uptake in the pancreas.

Thus it is helpful to be aware of what one expects to see (physiologic pattern and variants), what one is looking for (eg, a paraganglioma rather than a pheochromocytoma, a pulmonary carcinoid or a gastroenteropancreatic NET), where it should be localized (locoregional relapse or lymph nodes for MTC, adrenals for suspected pheochromocytoma, pancreas for insulinoma), how it is likely to appear (usually focal intense uptake that does not follow the physiologic biodistribution), and what could mask its identification (uptake in excretory organs such as gallbladder, pancreas, and urinary tract). Moreover, in recent years the introduction of hybrid PET/CT systems has offered another tool for the correct interpretation of areas of uptake, because CT images can be relied on for attenuation-corrected images that offer anatomic details which, in most cases, can localize anatomically the sites of ^{18}F-DOPA uptake.

Head and neck

^{18}F-DOPA is normally concentrated in the striatum while the rest of the brain shows no uptake of the tracer. In brain tumors the qualitative criterion used is that any tracer activity above the background level of adjacent brain can be considered abnormal. Standard visual analysis of ^{18}F-FDOPA PET seems adequate, with a high sensitivity in identifying tumor. However, the specificity is low because all radiation necrosis lesions have low but visible tracer uptake.[3] Therefore, different quantitative methods based on ratios between tumor and normal contralateral hemisphere (T/N), striatum (T/S), or white matter (T/W) can provide additional help. The specificity of ^{18}F-FDOPA in brain tumor imaging can be greatly increased by using a T/S threshold of 0.75 or 1.0, a T/N threshold of 1.3, or a T/W threshold of 1.6, which can help discriminate the pathologic area.[3] Using receiver-operator characteristic curves the optimal T/S threshold of greater than 1.0 for ^{18}F-DOPA shows sensitivity of 98%, specificity of 86%, positive predictive value of 95%, and negative predictive value of 95%. A recent study demonstrated that uptake is significantly higher in high-grade than in low-grade tumors in newly diagnosed (but not recurrent) tumors, and a

Table 2
Mean SUV$_{max}$ values of ^{18}F-DOPA physiologic accumulation in different organs with and without carbidopa

Organ	Mean SUV$_{max}$ in Adults			Mean SUV$_{max}$ in Children	
	Chondrogiannis et al,[51] 2012	Timmers et al,[40] 2007		Lopci et al,[41] 2012	
	No Carbidopa	No Carbidopa	Carbidopa	No Carbidopa	Carbidopa
Basal ganglia	2.77	2.43	3.73	2.1	3.4
Myocardium		2.53	3.18		
Lungs		0.69	0.88		
Liver	2.15	3.13	3.42	1.5	2.2
Kidneys	4.4	5.33	5.32	3.7	1.7
Gallbladder	8.5				
Pancreas		6.21	—	3.3	2.3
Pancreas uncinate process	5.67				
Pancreas body-tail region	4.1				
Bowel	2.3				
Bladder	111.9				
Adrenals	1.92				

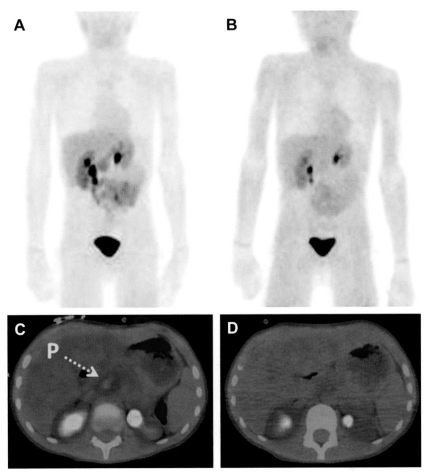

Fig. 2. 18F-DOPA PET/CT of an 8.5-year-old child with neuroblastoma. (*A, C*) Images without premedication with carbidopa (maximum-intensity projection [MIP] and transverse fused images). (*B, D*) Images after premedication with 50 mg carbidopa 1 hour before scanning. Note the uptake in the pancreas (*C, yellow arrow*) without carbidopa premedication, and the absent uptake owing to the effect of carbidopa administration (*D*). (*Courtesy of Egesta Lopci, MD, Bologna, Italy.*)

SUV_{max} of 2.72 was able to discriminate between low-grade and high-grade tumors, with sensitivity and specificity of 85% and 89%.[25] In the brain the only uptake of the tracer is seen in the striatum, which leaves it open to misinterpretation (**Fig. 3**).

Thorax
There is no confounding uptake in the thorax. Regarding the lungs, any focal uptake accompanied by a lesion on the CT images can be considered pathologic. Moreover, in the thorax the only structures that may present DOPA accumulation are the myocardium and the esophagus, which may show a mild uptake easily recognized as normal.

Abdomen and pelvis
18F-DOPA shows several sites of accumulation in the abdomen and pelvis region, mainly attributable to its excretory mechanisms: intense and variable uptake can be seen in the bile ducts, the gallbladder, and urinary pathways. A larger variability in 18F-DOPA uptake can be seen in the pancreas, especially in the uncinate process, which in some cases can show intense uptake. Similarly, uptake by the adrenal glands may be highly variable, and this must be taken into consideration to avoid misinterpretation of a normal adrenal as a pheochromocytoma (**Fig. 7**). When DOPA uptake, even if relatively high, is homogeneous, and is usually symmetric and not associated with morphologic alteration on CT imaging, the appearance should be considered as indicating normal adrenal uptake. No significant or mild diffuse uptake is usually noted in the bowel. As already mentioned, the excretory organs (gallbladder, kidneys, and urinary bladder) show a high variability in SUV_{max} values depending on individual elimination timing

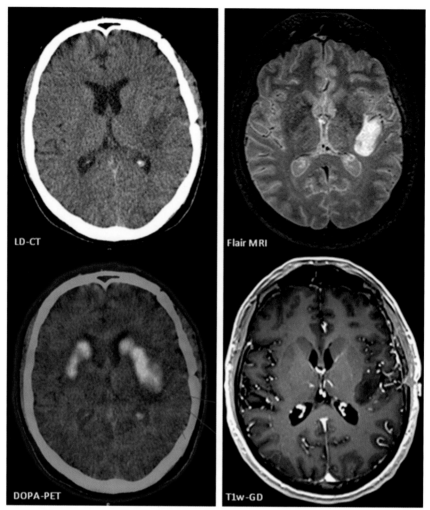

Fig. 3. A 41-year-old patient with an oligoastrocytoma II grade; MIB-1 3%. (*Upper left*) CT image. (*Upper right*) Fluid-attenuated inversion recovery (FLAIR) image. (*Lower left*) ^{18}F-DOPA PET/CT image. (*Lower right*) T1-weighted MR image. The uptake in the PET/CT image, even if close to the striatum, is unambiguously pathologic. In the brain the only site with normal uptake is the striatum, and only lesions close to the striatum could be misinterpreted. Note for MR imaging the typical behavior of low-grade gliomas: signal on FLAIR, and no enhancement after gadolinium contrast on T1-weighted image. (*Courtesy of* Egesta Lopci, MD, Bologna, Italy.)

and hydration status. The biodistribution data are relatively constant in terms of the intensity of liver uptake,[51] which could be helpful when semi-quantitative analyses based on the lesion-to-background ratio are needed. For this purpose, the liver uptake could be regarded as a background parameter.

On the other hand, in cases of suspicion of para-ganglioma/pheochromocytoma, any nonphysiologic extra-adrenal focal uptake or asymmetric adrenal uptake with a concordant enlarged gland, or adrenal uptake more intense than that of the liver with a concordant enlarged gland, can be considered pathologic.[48]

As already noted, premedication with carbidopa blocks physiologic tracer uptake by the pancreas

and can be a potential confounder in the detection of adrenal lesions.

POSSIBLE PITFALLS
Pitfalls Related to the Interpretation of PET and PET/CT Images

^{18}F-DOPA traces a very specific metabolic pathway and thus presents a very specific biodistribution pattern, which varies mainly as a result of variable excretion of the tracer through the excretory organs (**Table 3**).

In the head and neck region, the only possible pitfall can be provoked by a lesion located very close to the striatum, which is the only structure in the head that presents a significant uptake of

Table 3
Possible pitfalls with 18F-DOPA

Head and neck	Striatum	Physiologic uptake in the striatum could hide a possible brain tumor located close to it
Abdomen and pelvis	Gallbladder and biliary tract	Variable intense uptake in the gallbladder and the bile pathways could mimic an intestinal tumor or hepatic metastases
	Pancreas	1. Physiologic uptake in the pancreas could hide a pathologic area within the pancreatic parenchyma 2. Pancreatic uptake is a potential confounder in the detection of adrenal lesions (but can be prevented by blocking the pancreatic uptake by carbidopa)
	Urinary tract	1. Uptake in the kidneys could hide a pathologic uptake of the tail of the pancreas (left kidney); right kidney interferes less with the uncinate process of the pancreas 2. Uptake of the kidney could hide a pathologic uptake of the adrenals 3. Uptake in the ureters could resemble a pathologic abdominal uptake in the bowel or in lymph nodes. Misinterpretations could be avoided by performing late images after ambulation and/or hydration, or after diuretic administration

tracer. Uptake in the esophagus, oral cavity, myocardium, and mammary gland is so mild that it can be easily recognized as normal without confounding the physician.

On the other hand, the abdomen and pelvis region presents several sites with widely variable uptake that could confound the physician.

Gallbladder/Common bile duct

One of the major pitfalls presented by 18F-DOPA PET/CT is the intense focal uptake of the tracer in the gallbladder and, in some cases, the common bile duct; this could mimic an intestinal tumor or a hepatic metastasis from a neuroendocrine primary tumor, and has already been reported as a possible pitfall.[52] In this case, knowledge of the normal biodistribution of the tracer and its physiologic excretion through the biliary route, and the anatomic correlation offered by the coregistered CT images of the PET/CT scan, can help physicians identify easily the site of the uptake as physiologic activity in the gallbladder or the biliary path (**Figs. 4 and 5**).

Urinary excretion tract

Urinary excretion is the major excretion route of the tracer, and can be the cause of several pitfalls. The intense uptake of the tracer in the kidneys might mask pathologic uptake in the tail of the pancreas (left kidney); the activity in the right kidney interferes less with the head of the pancreas. Moreover, uptake in the kidneys could hide a pathologic uptake of the adrenals, especially in patients with dilatation of the superior caliceal groups or who present just an accumulation of

the tracer within the superior intrarenal urinary path. Uptake in the ureters, even if less intense and usually with a "spotted" appearance, might resemble pathologic abdominal uptake in the bowel, or lymph nodes. The bladder is less interfering, even if it presents an intense accumulation of the tracer, because usually a PET scan starts with an empty bladder. In all cases, besides the knowledge of the possible physiologic accumulation of the tracer, and always in relation to the clinical suspicion, the low-dose CT images for the attenuation correction of the hybrid PET/CT scanners offer the most important aid because they can precisely localize the anatomic counterpart of the uptake. Moreover, in cases of interpretative doubt the tracer (half-life of 110 minutes) offers the possibility to acquire late images after diuretic administration or after ambulation and hydration, which could alter the appearance of the uptake and help to discriminate between pathologic and physiologic (**Fig. 6**).

Pancreas

An obvious limitation of pancreatic PET imaging using 18F-DOPA is the physiologic uptake of tracer in pancreatic tissue. The physiologic intense and variable uptake in the pancreas can lead to 2 possible pitfalls: on the one hand, uptake in the pancreas, especially in the uncinate process, can be confused as a para-aortic pathologic lesion (false positive) and on the other, pancreas can contain a genuine lesion with the same uptake intensity not identified as pathologic by 18F-DOPA (false negative). Moreover, physiologic pancreatic uptake is a potential limitation of 18F-DOPA PET

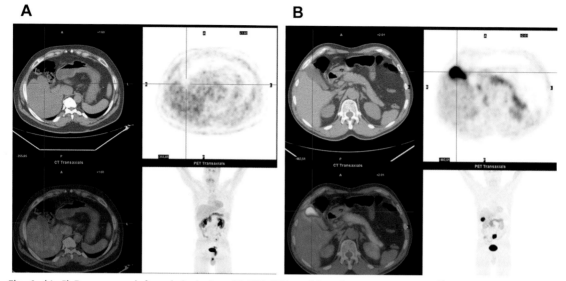

Fig. 4. (*A, B*) From upper left and clockwise: CT, PET, MIP, and fused PET/CT images of ^{18}F-DOPA PET/CT of 2 patients with absent (*A*) and very intense uptake (*B*) of ^{18}F-DOPA in the gallbladder that could mimic a liver or intestinal lesion. Note the variability in pancreas and kidney uptake in the 2 patients. Note also the mild diffuse uptake of the tracer in the intestinal loops, the myocardium and liver (*A, B*), the striatum, muscles, and oral cavity, as well as the ureters (*A*). The second patient presented an abdominal paraganglioma located just below the aortic carrefour. Images shown are without carbidopa premedication.

in the detection of adrenal lesions; in these cases premedication with carbidopa prevents masking of a possible lesion by blocking the pancreatic uptake. In addition, carbidopa not only "cleans" the vision in the peripancreatic region but also increases the uptake in the lesions, which thus can be more easily identified.

The utility of ^{18}F-DOPA PET/CT in adult patients with hyperinsulinemic hypoglycemia remains an open question in the literature, because the slight differences between pathologic or nonpathologic areas of the pancreas, which show a variable physiologic uptake of the tracer anyway, can be a possible pitfall. Moreover, premedication with carbidopa could lead to another possible methodological pitfall when considering patients with hyperinsulinemic hypoglycemia, because carbidopa (a peripheral AADC inhibitor) decreases the whole pancreatic uptake, decreasing also the lesion-to-background ratio.[40] Negativization of ^{18}F-DOPA focal pancreatic hot spots has been reported after premedication with carbidopa in patients with hyperinsulinemic hypoglycemia.[34,36,53,54]

Pitfalls Related to Pathology

Some possible sources of false-negative results of ^{18}F-DOPA PET/CT can be related to factors such as the small size of the lesion or tumor dedifferentiation. Genetic factors may also affect the ^{18}F-DOPA uptake in paragangliomas; SDHB gene

mutations may result in extra-adrenal paragangliomas for which ^{18}F-DOPA PET shows a lower sensitivity than for non–SDHB-related lesions.[31] On the other hand, the high specificity of ^{18}F-DOPA PET and PET/CT, explained by the fact that only neuroendocrine cells are able to take up, decarboxylate, and store amino acids and their amines, leads to few false-positive ^{18}F-DOPA PET findings.

Kauhanen and colleagues[2] described one patient with suspected paraganglioma recurrence and increased ^{18}F-DOPA uptake in the right adrenal; histologic verification showed a normal adrenal gland. Timmers and colleagues[55] reported one patient with a gastrointestinal stromal tumor that was visualized by ^{18}F-DOPA PET. Luster and colleagues[56] described an adrenal mass with a mildly intense ^{18}F-DOPA uptake, but clinical follow-up revealed no evidence of pheochromocytoma. However, when an adrenal mass presents a high or very high radiotracer uptake, a diagnosis of a pheochromocytoma is certain (**Fig. 7**).

Rischke and colleagues[57] reported 4 patients with false-positive results (of 33 patients studied) with ^{18}F-DOPA accumulation not specific for pheochromocytomas or paragangliomas that were verified by cross-sectional imaging and follow-up: (1) an anatomic variant of pancreas morphology, (2) diverticulum of duodenum, (3) moderate focal accumulation in paraesophageal tissue without evidence of nodular structure, and (4) moderate

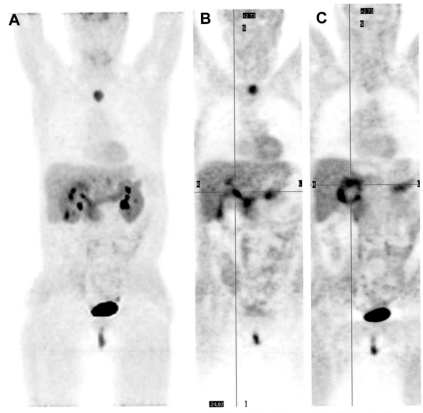

Fig. 5. ^{18}F-DOPA PET/CT of a 60-year-old female patient affected by Charcot-Marie-Tooth disease, already operated on, who presented with high calcitonin levels. (*A*) MIP image shows focal area of pathologic uptake in the thoracic inlet region suggestive for local relapse as well as an area of uptake in the left hepatic lobe. (*B, C*) Coronal PET images show physiologic uptake in the common biliary tract, gallbladder, and pancreas associated with a large area of intense pathologic uptake in the liver of maximum diameter of 5 cm, suggesting metastatic disease (*C*). Note the uptake in the right ureter (*C*) and in the liver, myocardium, bladder, and pancreas. Images shown are without carbidopa premedication.

focal accumulation in paracolic tissue without evidence of nodular structure.

Koopmans and colleagues[29] studied prospectively 53 patients with carcinoid tumor, and recorded a patient-based sensitivity of 100%, region-based sensitivity of 95%, and lesion-based sensitivity 96% better than CT, SRS, and combined CT/SRS, and did not report any false-positive case.

In a recent meta-analysis on MTC, investigators reported that false-positive findings with ^{18}F-DOPA are uncommon, but on the other hand that false-negative results might be related to small MTC lesions or dedifferentiation. In fact, comparative analysis of ^{18}F-DOPA and ^{18}F-FDG has shown better results with ^{18}F-DOPA in terms of sensitivity and specificity. These PET radiopharmaceuticals reflect 2 different metabolic pathways and seem to have a complementary role in recurrent MTC; a higher ^{18}F-DOPA uptake is related to a higher degree of cell differentiation, whereas a higher

FDG uptake is related to a poor differentiation/dedifferentiation. Based on literature findings, the diagnostic performance of ^{18}F-DOPA in recurrent MTC improved in patients with higher levels of serum calcitonin.[32,33] High levels of calcitonin and negative DOPA PET could depend on the small size of the recurrence. High levels of carcinoembryonic antigen and negative ^{18}F-DOPA PET could depend from dedifferentiation of the tumor and its inability to take up DOPA, so FDG would be the radiopharmaceutical of choice.

In an article by Tessonnier and colleagues,[34] the investigators report intense radiotracer uptake in the whole pancreas that was not statistically significant between controls (n = 37) and hyperinsulinemic patients (n = 6) with mean pancreatic SUV$_{max}$ 2.7 and 1.9, respectively; they conclude that ^{18}F-DOPA PET/CT seems to have a limited role in tumor localization in patients with hyperinsulinemic hypoglycemia. On the other hand, on

A

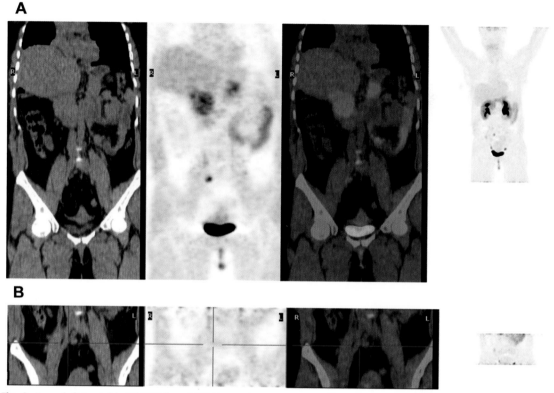

B

Fig. 6. From left to right: CT, PET, fused PET/CT, and MIP images of ¹⁸F-DOPA PET/CT scanning of a patient restaging for atypical pulmonary carcinoid tumor operated on in 2009. In 2012, liver metastases were surgically removed. The patient also underwent cholecystectomy. Whole-body PET/CT (*A*) revealed pathologic uptake on osteolytic areas on the skeleton. Moreover, a small area of focal uptake was seen in the upper pelvis in right paramedian region medially to what appeared to be the course of the right ureter. A late acquisition was performed (*B*) after ambulation and hydration at the focality disappeared, indicating radioactive urine in the right ureter. Note the absent DOPA uptake in the gallbladder (cholecystectomy). Images shown are without carbidopa premedication.

the same topic Kauhanen and colleagues[4] report excellent results in 9 of 10 patients, reporting mean SUV_{max} in the affected pancreas of 4.4 versus mean SUV_{max} of 3.2 in other parts of the pancreas. Possible masking of a pheochromocytoma could be prevented by blockade of pancreatic uptake by carbidopa. Other pitfalls of ¹⁸F-DOPA PET of paraganglioma include tracer accumulation in the gallbladder and renal collecting system, mimicking an extra-adrenal tumor.[40] False-positive results may be related to tracer uptake by other neuroendocrine lesions. Rarely, uptake may be due to nonspecific inflammation (pneumonia, postoperative changes), as high levels of amino acid transport have also been found in macrophages. False negatives may include small lesions and abdominal SDH-mutation–related paragangliomas.[33,48]

In the brain the list of nontumoral uptake of all radiolabeled amino acids is also long, and includes ischemic brain areas, infarction, scar tissue, abscess, sarcoidosis, irradiated areas, hemangioma,

and many other nonneoplastic processes. Active inflammatory cells also require amino acids, and the increased perfusion of infections may contribute even further to the uptake of amino acids.

Technical Pitfalls

PET-CT represents a major technological advance, consisting of 2 complementary modalities that provide both functional and anatomic information and whose combined strength tends to overcome their respective weaknesses. With combined PET/CT, the superimposition of the precise structural findings provided by CT allows an accurate correlation of the radiotracer activity seen at PET with the correct anatomic or pathologic equivalent. When attenuation correction is based on the CT images there is a potential risk of overestimating the true activity of the tracer, as in the case of photopenic areas corresponding

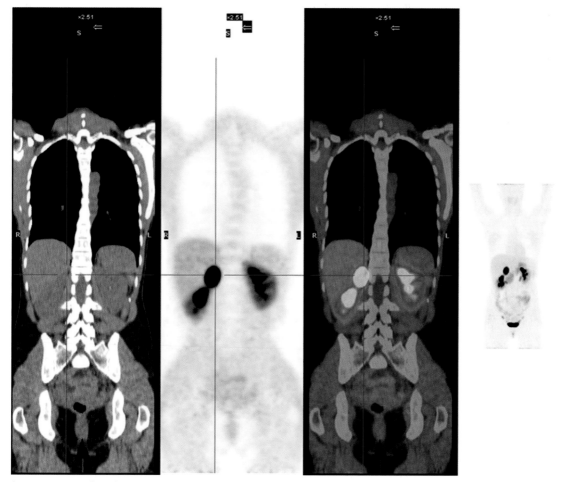

Fig. 7. A young female patient (39 years old) with hypertension and high levels of urinary normetanephrine. From left to right: Coronal images of CT, PET, fused PET/CT, and MIP images of ¹⁸F-DOPA PET/CT scan shows a large ovoidal area of very intense pathologic uptake (SUV_{max} 40.0) in the right adrenal (maximum diameter 3.5 cm), suggesting pheochromocytoma. Images shown are without carbidopa premedication.

to high-density structures on CT (metallic implants, surgical clips, barium).[58]

Another possible pitfall result from misregistration between PET and CT images; thus a superimposition of radiotracer activity on the wrong anatomic structure seen at CT, which can be due to breathing, patient motion, bowel motility, and so forth, can cause false-positive or false-negative PET findings.

SUMMARY

¹⁸F-DOPA is a radiopharmaceutical with interesting clinical applications and promising performances in the evaluation of the integrity of dopaminergic pathways, brain tumors, NETs (especially MTCs, paragangliomas, and pheochromocytomas), and congenital hyperinsulinism. ¹⁸F-DOPA traces a very specific metabolic pathway and has a very precise biodistribution pattern. As for any radiopharmaceutical, the knowledge of the normal distribution of ¹⁸F-DOPA, its physiologic variants, and its possible pitfalls is essential for the correct interpretation of PET scans. Moreover, it is important to be aware of the potential false-positive and false-negative episodes that can occur in the various clinical settings.

ACKNOWLEDGMENTS

The authors would like to thank Dr Egesta Lopci, Laura Evangelista, Karel Pacak, and Elise Blanchet for the images and the useful information provided.

REFERENCES

1. Nanni C, Fantini L, Nicolini S, et al. Non FDG PET. Clin Radiol 2010;65:536–48.

2. Kauhanen A, Seppanen M, Ovaska J, et al. The clinical value of [18F]fluoro-dihydroxyphenylalanine positron emission tomography in primary diagnosis, staging, and restaging of neuroendocrine tumors. Endocr Relat Cancer 2009;16:255–65.

3. Chen W. Clinical applications of PET in brain tumors. J Nucl Med 2007;48(9):1468–81.

4. Kauhanen S, Seppänen M, Minn H, et al. Fluorine-18-L-dihydroxyphenylalanine (18F-DOPA) positron emission tomography as a tool to localize an insulinoma or beta-cell hyperplasia in adult patients. J Clin Endocrinol Metab 2007;92(4):1237–44.

5. Mohnike K, Blakenstein O, Minn H, et al. [18F]-DOPA positron emission tomography for preoperative localization in congenital hyperinsulinism. Horm Res 2008;70(2):65–72.

6. Caroli P, Nanni C, Rubello D, et al. Non-FDG PET in the practice of oncology. Indian J Cancer 2010;47: 120–5.

7. Kao CH, Hsu WL, Xie HL, et al. GMP production of [18F]FDOPA and issue concerning its quality analyses as in USP 'Fluorodopa F 18 Injection'. Ann Nucl Med 2011;25:309–16.

8. Jager PL, Chirakal R, Marriott CJ, et al. 6-L-18F-Fluorodihydroxyphenylalanine PET in neuroendocrine tumors: basic aspects and emerging clinical applications. J Nucl Med 2008;49:573–86.

9. Fluorodopa F18 (Systemic). Available at: http://www.drugs.com. Accessed October 11, 2013.

10. Luxen A, Guillaume M, Melega WP, et al. Production of 6-[18F]Fluoro-L-DOPA and its metabolism in vivo: critical review. Int J Rad Appl Instrum B 1992;19:149–58.

11. Wahl L, Nahmias C. Modeling of fluorine-18-6-fluoro-L-dopa in humans. J Nucl Med 1996;37: 432–7.

12. Firnau G, Gernett ES, Chirakal R, et al. [18F]Fluoro-L-DOPA for the in vivo study of intracerebral dopamine. Int J Rad Appl Instrum A 1986;37:669–75.

13. Brouwers AH, Koopmans KP, Dierckx RA, et al. DOPA PET/CT. In: Fanti S, Farsad M, Mansi L, editors. PET/CT beyond FDG: a quick guide to image interpretation, Chapter 10. Heidelberg (Germany): Springer; 2010. p. 161–79.

14. Leenders KL, Salmon EP, Tyrrell P, et al. The nigrostriatal dopaminergic system assessed in vivo by positron emission tomography in healthy volunteer subjects and patients with Parkinson's disease. Arch Neurol 1990;47:1290–8.

15. Eidelberg D. Positron emission tomography studies in parkinsonism. Neurol Clin 1992;10:421–33.

16. Sawle GV. The detection of pre-clinical Parkinson's disease: what is the role of positron emission tomography? Mov Disord 1993;8:271–7.

17. Eshuis SA, Maguire RP, Leenders KL, et al. Comparison of 123I-FP-CIT SPECT with F-DOPA PET in patients with de novo and advanced Parkinson's disease. Eur J Nucl Med Mol Imaging 2006;33: 200–9.

18. Heiss WD, Wienhard K, Wagner R, et al. F-Dopa as an amino acid tracer to detect brain tumors. J Nucl Med 1996;37:1180–2.

19. Ishiwata K, Kutota K, Murakami M, et al. Re-evaluation of amino acid PET studies: can the protein synthesis rates in brain and tumor tissues be measured in vivo? J Nucl Med 1993;34:1936–43.

20. Jager PL, Vaalburg W, Pruim J, et al. Radiolabeled amino acids: basic aspects and clinical applications in oncology. J Nucl Med 2001;42:432–45.

21. Isselbacher KJ. Sugar and amino acid transport by cells in culture: differences between normal and malignant cells. N Engl J Med 1972;286:929–33.

22. Busch H, Davis JR, Honig GR, et al. The uptakes of a variety of amino acids into nuclear proteins of tumors and other tissues. Cancer Res 1959;19: 1030–9.

23. Sasajima T, Miyagawa T, Oku T, et al. Proliferation-dependent changes in amino acid transport and glucose metabolism in glioma cell lines. Eur J Nucl Med Mol Imaging 2004;31:1244–56.

24. Roelcke U, Radu EW, von Ammon K, et al. Alteration of blood-brain barrier in human brain tumors: comparison of [18F]fluorodeoxyglucose, [11C] methionine and rubidium-82 using PET. J Neurol Sci 1995;132:20–7.

25. Fueger BJ, Czernin J, Cloughesy T, et al. Correlation of 6-18F-fluoro-L-dopa PET uptake with proliferation and tumor grade in newly diagnosed and recurrent gliomas. J Nucl Med 2010;51:1532–8.

26. Walter F, Cloughesy T, Walter MA, et al. Impact of 3,4-dihydroxy-6-18F-fluoro-L-phenylalanine PET/CT on managing patients with brain tumors: the referring physician's perspective. J Nucl Med 2012; 53(3):393–8.

27. Nanni C, Fanti S, Rubello D. 18F-DOPA PET and PET/CT. J Nucl Med 2007;48(10):1577–9.

28. Pacak K, Eisenhofer G, Goldstein DS. Functional imaging of endocrine tumors: role of positron emission tomography. Endocr Rev 2004;25:568–80.

29. Koopmans KP, de Vries EG, Kema IP, et al. Staging of carcinoid tumours with 18F-DOPA PET: a prospective, diagnostic accuracy study. Lancet Oncol 2006;7(9):728–34.

30. Solcia E, Kloppel G, Sobin L. Histological typing of the endocrine tumours. 2nd edition. Berlin: Springer; 2000.

31. Treglia G, Cocciolillo F, de Waure C, et al. Diagnostic performance of 18F-dihydroxyphenylalanine positron emission tomography in patients with paraganglioma: a meta-analysis. Eur J Nucl Med Mol Imaging 2012;39(7):1144–53.

32. Treglia G, Cocciolillo F, Di Nardo F, et al. Detection rate of recurrent medullary thyroid carcinoma using fluorine-18 dihydroxyphenylalanine positron

emission tomography: a meta-analysis. Acad Radiol 2012;19(10):1290–9.

33. Marzola MC, Pelizzo MR, Ferdeghini M, et al. Dual PET/CT with (18)F-DOPA and (18)F-FDG in metastatic medullary thyroid carcinoma and rapidly increasing calcitonin levels: comparison with conventional imaging. Eur J Surg Oncol 2010;36: 414–21.

34. Tessonnier L, Sebag F, Ghander C, et al. Limited value of 18F-F-DOPA PET to localize pancreatic insulin-secreting tumors in adults with hyperinsulinemic hypoglycemia. J Clin Endocrinol Metab 2010;95(1):303–7.

35. Hardy O, Hernandez-Pampaloni M, Saffer JR, et al. Diagnosis and localization of focal congenital hyperinsulinism by 18F-fluorodopa PET scan. J Pediatr 2007;150:140–5.

36. de Lonlay P, Simon-Carre A, Ribeiro MJ, et al. Congenital hyperinsulinism: pancreatic [18F]fluoro-L-dihydroxyphenylalanine (DOPA) positron emission tomography and immunohistochemistry study of DOPA decarboxylase and insulin secretion. J Clin Endocrinol Metab 2006;91(3):933–40.

37. Jaffe M. Qinical studies of carbidopa and L-DOPA in the treatment of Parkinson's disease. Adv Neurol 1973;2:161.

38. Pinder RM, Brogden RN, Sawyer PW, et al. Levodopa and decarboxylase inhibitors: a review of their clinical pharmacology and use in the treatment of parkinsonism. Drugs 1976;11(5):329–77.

39. Brown WD, Oakes TR, DeJesus OT, et al. Fluorine-18-fluoro-L-DOPA dosimetry with carbidopa pretreatment. J Nucl Med 1998;39:1884–91.

40. Timmers HJ, Hadi M, Carrasquillo JA, et al. The effects of carbidopa on uptake of 6-18F-Fluoro-L-DOPA in PET of pheochromocytoma and extraadrenal abdominal paraganglioma. J Nucl Med 2007; 48(10):1599–606.

41. Lopci E, D'Ambrosio D, Nanni C, et al. Feasibility of carbidopa premedication in pediatric patients: a pilot study. Cancer Biother Radiopharm 2012; 27(10):729–33.

42. Mohnike K, Blankenstein O, Christesen HT, et al. Proposal for a standardized protocol for 18F-DOPA-PET (PET/CT) in congenital hyperinsulinism. Horm Res 2006;66:40–2.

43. Grassetto G, Massaro A, Cittadin S, et al. Kinetic of 18F-DOPA in basal ganglia of non-human primate. Eur J Nucl Med Mol Imaging 2009;35(Suppl 2): 145–539.

44. Koopmans KP, Brouwers AH, De Hooge MN, et al. Carcinoid crisis after injection of 6-18F-fluorodihydroxyphenylalanine in a patient with metastatic carcinoid. J Nucl Med 2005;46:1240–3.

45. Schiesser M, Veit-Haibach P, Muller MK, et al. Value of combined 6-[18F]fluorodihydroxyphenylalanine

PET/CT for imaging of neuroendocrine tumours. Br J Surg 2010;97(5):691–7.

46. Lovenberg W, Weissbach H, Undenfriend S. Aromatic L-amino acid decarboxylase. J Biol Chem 1962;237:89–93.

47. Treglia G, Rufini V, Salvatori M, et al. PET imaging in recurrent medullary thyroid carcinoma. Int J Mol Imaging 2012;2012:324686. http://dx.doi.org/10.1155/2012/324686.

48. Taïeb D, Timmers HJ, Hindié E, et al. EANM 2012 guidelines for radionuclide imaging of phaeochromocytoma and paraganglioma. Eur J Nucl Med Mol Imaging 2012;39(12):1977–95.

49. Beheshti M, Pocher S, Vali R, et al. The value of 18F-DOPA PET-CT in patients with medullary thyroid carcinoma: comparison with 18F-FDG PETCT. Eur Radiol 2009;19:1425–34.

50. Soussan M, Nataf V, Kerrou K, et al. Added value of early 18F-FDOPA PET/CT acquisition time in medullary thyroid cancer. Nucl Med Commun 2012;33: 775–9.

51. Chondrogiannis S, Grassetto G, Marzola MC, et al. 18F-DOPA PET/CT biodistribution consideration in 107 consecutive patients with neuroendocrine tumours. Nucl Med Commun 2012;33(2):179–84.

52. Balan KK. Visualization of the gall bladder on F-18 FDOPA PET imaging: a potential pitfall. Clin Nucl Med 2005;30(1):23–4.

53. Ribeiro MJ, De Lonlay P, Delzescaux T, et al. Characterization of hyperinsulinism in infancy assessed with PET and 18F-fluoro-L-DOPA. J Nucl Med 2005; 46:560–6.

54. Kauhanen S, Seppänen M, Nuutila P. Premedication with carbidopa masks positive finding of insulinoma and β-cell hyperplasia in [(18)F]-dihydroxy-phenylalanine positron emission tomography. J Clin Oncol 2008;26:5307–8 [author reply: 5308–9].

55. Timmers HJ, Chen CC, Carrasquillo JA, et al. Comparison of 18F-fluoro-L-DOPA, 18Ffluoro-deoxyglucose, and 18F-fluorodopamine PET and 123IMIBG scintigraphy in the localization of pheochromocytoma and paraganglioma. J Clin Endocrinol Metab 2009;94:4757–67.

56. Luster M, Karges W, Zeich K, et al. Clinical value of 18F-fluorodihydroxyphenylalanine positron emission tomography/computed tomography (18F-DOPA PET/CT) for detecting pheochromocytoma. Eur J Nucl Med Mol Imaging 2010;37:484–93.

57. Rischke HC, Benz MR, Wild D, et al. Correlation of the genotype of paragangliomas and pheochromocytomas with their metabolic phenotype on 3,4-dihydroxy-6-18F-fluoro-L-phenylalanin PET. J Nucl Med 2012;53(9):1352–8.

58. Blake MA, Singh A, Setty BN, et al. Pearls and pitfalls in interpretation of abdominal and pelvic PET-CT. Radiographics 2006;26(5):1335–53.

The Use of Gallium-68 Labeled Somatostatin Receptors in PET/CT Imaging

Valentina Ambrosini, MD, PhD*, Cristina Nanni, MD,
Stefano Fanti, MD

KEYWORDS

- 68Ga-DOTA-SSTRTs • PET/CT • Neuroendocrine tumors • Somatostatin receptors

KEY POINTS

- 68Ga-DOTA-SSTRTs PET/computed tomography (CT) is the most promising noninvasive imaging procedure to study well-differentiated neuroendocrine tumors (NET).
- 68Ga-DOTA-SSTRTs specifically bind to somatostatin receptors (SSTR) subtypes overexpressed on NET cells (with variable affinity) but at present there are no clinical reports supporting the preferential use of one analogue (DOTA-TOC, DOTA-NOC, DOTA-TATE) over the other.
- 68Ga-DOTA-SSTRTs' accuracy in NET lesions detection is superior to morphologic imaging procedures, SRS, and PET/CT with metabolic tracers (18F-FDG, 18F-DOPA).
- Causes of false positive reporting include accessory spleens, inflammation, and lymphoma.
- Causes of false negative reporting include small lesions size and variable/absent SSTR expression.
- PET/CT with 68Ga-DOTA-SSTRTs has a relevant impact on a patient's clinical management (in particular, regarding the choice of the treatment plan) and provides prognostic information.

INTRODUCTION

Clinical Background

Somatostatin receptors (SSTR) are G-coupled proteins widely distributed in the human body, and 5 different receptor subtypes have been described in humans. SSTR are the molecular target of several radiotracers for neuroendocrine tumor (NET) imaging.

In fact, a few decades ago, the introduction in the clinic of somatostatin receptor scintigraphy (SRS) completely changed the diagnostic approach to NET. This procedure showed an overall detection rate of SSTR-positive tumors[1] ranging between 80% and 100%. More recently, new β-emitting radiotracers (68Ga-DOTA-SSTRTs) have been developed and are increasingly used in Europe for NET imaging as part of clinical trials. The employment of PET/computed tomography (CT) allows the well-known limitation of SRS to be overcome, such as a lower spatial resolution (due to suboptimal spatial resolution of the isotopes used for single-photon emission computerized tomography [SPECT] imaging),[2,3] the relatively higher costs (as compared with PET imaging), the longer image acquisition protocol, and a better visualization of organs with higher octreotide-physiologic uptake (eg, liver).

68Ga-DOTA-SSTRTs present a common structure: a β-emitting isotope (68Ga), a chalet (DOTA), and the ligand of SSTR (NOC, TOC, TATE). Currently, several different compounds have been used (DOTA-TOC, DOTA-NOC, DOTA-TATE) with variable affinity for SSTR subtypes: all radiotracers can bind to SSTR2 and to SSTR5, whereas only 68Ga-DOTA-NOC presents a good affinity for SSTR3.[4–6]

The encouraging results obtained with 68Ga-DOTA-SSTRTs PET/CT in NET patients determined the exponential increase of their employment in

Conflict of Interest: The authors state that they have nothing to disclose.
Nuclear Medicine, S.Orsola-Malpighi University Hospital, via Massarenti 9, Bologna 40138, Italy
* Corresponding author. Nuclear Medicine, S.Orsola-Malpighi University Hospital, University of Bologna, Pad 30, Via Massarenti 9, Bologna 40138, Italy.
E-mail address: valentina.ambrosini@aosp.bo.it

PET Clin 9 (2014) 323–329
http://dx.doi.org/10.1016/j.cpet.2014.03.008
1556-8598/14/$ – see front matter © 2014 Elsevier Inc. All rights reserved.

several centers. The first compound that has been used in humans was DOTA-TOC, followed by DOTA-NOC and DOTA-TATE. The overall sensitivity and specificity of 68Ga-DOTA-SSTRTs for the detection of NET range between 90% to 98% and 92% to 98%, respectively.[7,8]

Current guidelines state that there is no evidence supporting the preferential use of one analogue over the other[9] and recent papers of comparison reported comparable diagnostic accuracy.[10,11] Factors in favor of the use of DOTA-NOC include the wider spectrum of SSTR affinity and lower dosimetry, whereas both DOTA-TOC and DOTA-TATE have the advantage that they can be used for diagnosis (if labeled with 68Ga) and subsequent treatment (when labeled with Lutetium 177 [177Lu] or Yttrium 90 [90Y]).

68Ga-DOTA-SSTRTs present several advantages as compared with other PET tracers to study NET. One of the technical advantages of 68Ga-DOTA-SSTRTs is certainly the easy and economic synthesis and labeling process: gallium can be easily eluted from a commercially available Ge68/Ga68 generator and therefore there is no need of an on-site cyclotron. Gallium 68 ($t_{1/2}$ = 68 min) presents an 89% positron emission and negligible γ-emission (1077 keV) of 3.2%. The long half-life of the mother radionuclide germanium 68 (68Ge; 270.8 days) makes it possible to use the generator for approximately 9 to 12 months depending on the requirement, rendering the whole procedure relatively economic. Another advantage of 68Ga-SSTRTs in comparison to metabolic tracers (eg, 18F-DOPA, 18F-FDG) is that they provide data on receptors expression, particularly relevant before starting targeted nuclide therapy. Finally, as compared with SRS, PET/CT is a single-day examination.

The indication to perform PET/CT in NET patients includes disease staging/restaging, follow-up, detection of unknown primary tumor sites, and selection of candidates who might benefit from therapy with either hot or cold somatostatin analogues.

Several reports described the good results obtained by using 68Ga-DOTA-SSTRTs for the detection of NET (**Fig. 1**), including small lesions at different anatomic sites. It is now well known that 68Ga-DOTA-SSTRTs PET/CT is more accurate for the detection of well-differentiated NET lesions than CT, SRS, and even PET/CT performed using metabolic tracers (such as 18F-FDG and 18F-DOPA).

One of the studies with the largest populations (84 patients)[7] demonstrated that 68Ga-DOTA-TOC PET/CT accuracy (96%) was significantly higher than that of CT (75%) and Indium 111 SRS-SPECT (58%). PET/CT was particularly accurate for the detection of lesions at the node, bone, and liver level. Overall, PET/CT-derived data were relevant to change the patient's clinical management in 14% of the cases when compared with SPECT and in 21% when compared with CT. A more recent paper comparing 68Ga-DOTA-TATE PET/CT with SRS reported that in patients with negative or weakly positive findings on SRS PET/CT documented 168 versus 28 lesions.[12]

In addition, 68Ga-DOTA-SSTRTs showed promise in better determination of the patient's

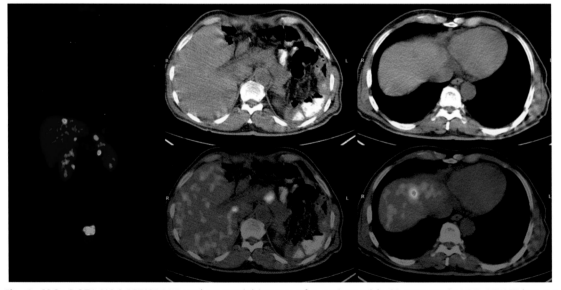

Fig. 1. 68Ga-DOTA-NOC PET/CT MIP and transaxial images of a patient with G2 pancreatic NET. PET/CT images show the presence of increased tracer uptake (SUVmax 56) at pancreatic (body) and liver (2 focal areas) level.

clinical management[13]: 68Ga-DOTA-NOC PET/CT findings affected either stage classification or therapy modifications in half the patients of a population of 90 cases with biopsy-proven NET.

The radiotracer/receptor interaction justifies the employment of PET/CT to have information on SSTR expression on NET cells. In fact, the possibility of acquiring these data in a noninvasive manner is certainly very appealing for the clinicians, both because it can provide an indirect measure of cell differentiation[14,15] and because it can guide the choice of the most appropriate treatment option.

Lesions with a high 68Ga-DOTA-peptide uptake have a higher differentiation grade, have a lower growth rate, are more likely to respond to treatment with either hot or cold somatostatin analogues, and are therefore associated with a better prognosis.[14] In fact, semiquantitative and visual interpretation of 68Ga-DOTA-SSTRT uptake is used to guide the quantity of radiation and the timing for targeted radionuclide therapy, using either 177Lu or 90YDOTA-TOC. At present 68Ga-DOTA-SSTRTs PET/CT is used as a baseline procedure before starting target treatment with somatostatin analogues. However, its clinical impact in the assessment of treatment response is under debate and 18F-DOPA seems to be more suitable for the therapy monitoring. Detection of primary tumor in patients with biopsy-proven NET metastases is another common indication of 68Ga-DOTA-SSTRTs PET/CT.[16]

Few studies directly compared the diagnostic performance of 68Ga-DOTA-SSTRTs with metabolic tracers. In particular, 68Ga-DOTA-SSTRTs were reported to be more accurate than 18F-DOPA in well-differentiated NETs.[17,18] Moreover, the easy and economic synthesis process, in addition to the fact that 68Ga-DOTA-SSTRTs also provide data on SSTR expression, is in favor of the use of these compounds as compared with 18F-DOPA.

On the contrary, NET forms showing absent or variable SSTR expression (eg, medullar thyroid carcinoma, neuroblastoma) or NET arising at sites of known physiologic 68Ga-DOTA-SSTRTs uptake (eg, adrenals) are better investigated with 18F-DOPA.

In cases presenting a low differentiation grade or variable/absent SSTR expression, 18F-FDG may offer both diagnostic and prognostic information: the detection of highly metabolic lesions is associated with a worse outcome.[19]

68Ga-DOTA-SSTRTs PET/CT Imaging

The European Association of Nuclear Medicine recently published guidelines for 68Ga-DOTA-SSTRTs PET/CT image acquisition and image interpretation.[9] Gallium 68 may be eluted from a commercially available 68Ge/68Ga generator and the labeling of the DOTA-peptide with 68Ga is performed following standard procedures using semi-automated or fully automated systems. They are based on either prepurification and concentration of the generator eluate using and anion-exchange[20,21] or cation-exchange technique,[22] or they use a fraction of the generator eluate directly for radiolabeling.[23,24] Radiolabeling is performed using a suitable buffer at elevated temperature followed by chromatographic purification of the radiolabeling solution using a C-18 cartridge and an appropriate aseptic formulation. The method used ensures a level of 68Ge in the final preparation lower than 0.001% of the 68Ga radioactivity. Quality control protocols include tests for radionuclide purity, radiochemical purity (high-performance liquid chromatography, thin layer chromatography), chemical purity (buffer, solvents), and sterility and endotoxin testing using validated methods.[9]

PET/CT imaging is performed following the intravenous administration of approximately 100 MBq (75–250 MBq) of the radiolabeled peptide (68Ga-DOTA-NOC, DOTA-TOC, DOTA-TATE). It is to be noted that no specific patient's preparation

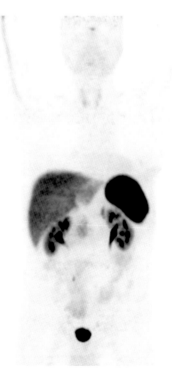

Fig. 2. 68Ga-DOTA-NOC physiologic biodistribution. Physiologic uptake areas include the pituitary gland, the spleen, the liver, the adrenal glands, the head of the pancreas, the thyroid (very mild uptake), and the urinary tract (kidneys and urinary bladder).

is warranted before scanning. In particular, no fasting nor discontinuation of somatostatin analogues treatment is required before imaging.[9] Patients are encouraged to void before image acquisition to reduce the background noise as well as the radiation dose to kidneys and bladder.

Images are generally acquired after an uptake time of 60 minutes (45–90 min).

Finally, the employment of contrast media is not recommended for routine scanning.[25]

While interpreting 68Ga-DOTA-SSTRTs PET/CT images, it is important to consider the tracer biodistribution first (Fig. 2). Physiologic uptake areas include the pituitary gland, the spleen, the liver, the adrenal glands, the head of the pancreas, the thyroid (very mild uptake), and the urinary tract (kidneys and urinary bladder).

Several conditions may account for false positive reporting. First of all, because SSTR are expressed on activated lymphocytes, both inflammatory conditions and lymphoma are associated with increased 68Ga-DOTA-SSTRTs uptake (Figs. 3 and 4). Particular care should be devoted to the interpretation of areas that are frequent sites

of inflammation, such as thyroid, mediastinal nodes, inguinal nodes, and nodes adjacent to areas of recent surgery/trauma. A detailed clinical history with particular attention to concomitant disorders (eg, sarcoidosis, chronic gastritis, chronic thryoiditis) and recent invasive procedures or trauma may often help image interpretation.

A quite common benign condition that can be challenging for the reporting physician is the presence of uptake in the head of the pancreas (exocrine). Gabriel and colleagues[7] were the first to report this condition in 67.8% of the 80 cases studied with 68Ga-DOTA-TOC. Benign uptake in the head of the pancreas was also reported using 68Ga-DOTA-NOC in 36% of the studied cases: the diffuse uptake pattern (23%) was more frequent than the focal (8%).[26]

Finally another benign condition that can be associated with false positive reporting is the presence of accessory spleens.

Considering that the uptake of 68Ga-DOTA-SSTRTs depends on the presence of SSTR on NET cells, tumors with low, variable, or absent receptor expression may result falsely negative.

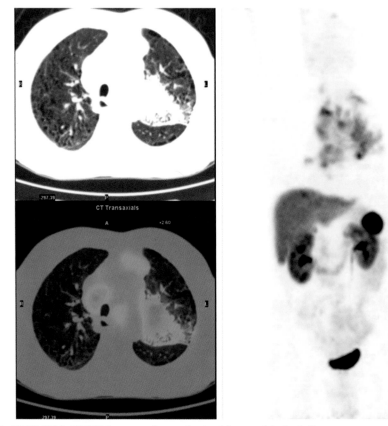

Fig. 3. 68Ga-DOTA-NOC PET/CT images of a patient with sarcoidosis. Inflammatory processes show increased tracer uptake and may represent a cause of false positive reporting.

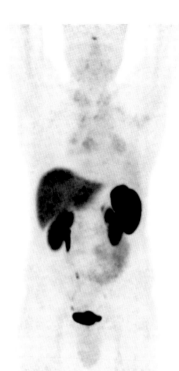

Fig. 4. 68Ga-DOTA-NOC PET/CT images of a patient with lymphoma. Activated lymphocytes present SSTR expression and may be visualized on 68Ga-DOTA-NOC PET/CT images, representing a possible cause of false positive reporting.

Histologic tumor types that fall into this category include medullary thyroid carcinoma, neuroblastoma, insulinoma, and pheocromocytoma. Of course, low-grade NET and lesions smaller than PET spatial resolution (5 mm) may also account for false negative reporting.

EFFECTS OF TREATMENT ON 68GA-DOTA-PEPTIDES UPTAKE

Although a potential effect of somatostatin analogues on tracer uptake was hypothesized, current guidelines do not recommend withdrawal before image acquisition.[9]

EFFECTS OF AGING ON 68GA-DOTA-PEPTIDES UPTAKE

To the authors' knowledge, there are no reports in the literature describing the effect of aging on SSTR expression and consequently on 68Ga-DOTA-peptides uptake.

PHYSIOLOGIC UPTAKE, BENIGN FINDINGS, AND PITFALLS

1. Head and neck
   Physiologic uptake: pituitary, thyroid (very mild)
   Benign findings: chronic thyroiditis, thyroid nodules, inflammation/infection secondary to trauma or surgery
   False negative findings: lesions less than 5 mm, medullary thyroid cancer (some forms)
2. Thorax
   Physiologic uptake: no
   Benign findings: inflammatory/infectious thoracic disorders (pneumonia, granulomatous disorders, lung fibrosis), inflammation/infection secondary to trauma or surgery
   False negative findings: lesions less than 5 mm, neuroblastoma
3. Abdomen and pelvis
   Physiologic uptake: head of the pancreas, adrenals, liver, spleen, intestine, urinary tract (kidneys, ureters, urinary bladder), mildly diffuse uptake in the prostate
   Benign findings: accessory spleen, inflammatory/infectious abdominal disorders (eg, pancreatitis, chronic gastritis), inflammation/infection secondary to trauma or surgery
   False negative findings: lesions less than 5 mm, benign insulinoma, neuroblastoma, pheocromocytoma

SUMMARY

68Ga-DOTA-SSTRTs PET/CT has become the most promising noninvasive procedure to study well-differentiated NET. Although the excellent diagnostic accuracy of the procedure is well known, its use is limited to specialized centers in Europe as parts of clinical trials. Literature reports confirm the superiority of 68Ga-DOTA-SSTRTs PET/CT for the assessment of well-differentiated NET over morphologic imaging procedures, SRS, and even PET/CT using metabolic radiotracers. 68Ga-DOTA-SSTRTs provide good visualization of NET lesions at both the primary and the metastatic sites (node, bone, liver, and unusual localizations).

The advantages of their use over metabolic tracers (18F-DOPA, 18F-FDG) are not only limited to a better overall detection rate but also to the fact that they also provide data on SSTR expression on target lesions, resulting a fundamental procedure before starting therapy with either hot or cold somatostatin analogues. Moreover, they can be used also in centers without an on-site cyclotron.

To interpret 68Ga-DOTA-SSTRTs images correctly, it is crucial to understand the tracer's biodistribution as well as the conditions that may alter tracer uptake. Considering that SSTR are expressed on activated lymphocytes, all areas of inflammation show 68Ga-DOTA-SSTRTs uptake. Areas of increased uptake in frequent sites of inflammation (eg, thyroid, mediastinal nodes, inguinal nodes, and nodes adjacent to areas of recent surgery/trauma) should be interpreted with care. A detailed clinical history with particular attention to concomitant disorders (eg, sarcoidosis, chronic gastritis, chronic thryoiditis) and recent invasive procedures or trauma may often help image interpretation. The presence of uptake in the head of the pancreas should always be carefully evaluated because it may often be benign. Otherwise, because the pancreas is also a frequent site of NET onset, particular attention should be devoted to the evaluation of the uptake pattern (diffuse more likely to be benign) and to the comparison with other imaging techniques.

REFERENCES

1. Krenning EP, Kwekkeboom DJ, Bakker WH, et al. Somatostatin receptor scintigraphy with [111In-DTPA-D-Phe1]-and [123I-Tyr3]-octreotide: the Rotterdam experience with more than 1000 patients. Eur J Nucl Med 1993;20:716–31.

2. Kowalski J, Henze M, Schuhmacher J, et al. Evaluation of positron emission tomography imaging using [68Ga]-DOTA-D-Phe1-Tyr3-octreotide in comparison to [111In]-DTPAOC SPECT. First results in patients with neuroendocrine tumors. Mol Imaging Biol 2003;5:42–8.

3. Buchmann I, Henze M, Engelbrecht S, et al. Comparison of 68Ga-DOTATOC PET and 111In-DTPAOC (Octreoscan) SPECT in patients with neuroendocrine tumours. Eur J Nucl Med Mol Imaging 2007; 34(10):1617–26.

4. Antunes P, Ginj M, Zhang H, et al. Are radiogallium-labelled DOTA-conjugated somatostatin analogues superior to those labelled with other radiometals? Eur J Nucl Med Mol Imaging 2007;34(7):982–93.

5. Reubi JC. Peptide receptors as molecular targets for cancer diagnosis and therapy. Endocr Rev 2003; 24(4):389–427.

6. Reubi JC, Waser B. Concomitant expression of several peptide receptors in neuroendocrine tumours: molecular basis for in vivo multireceptor tumour targeting. Eur J Nucl Med Mol Imaging 2003; 30(5):781–93.

7. Gabriel M, Decristoforo C, Kendler D, et al. 68Ga-DOTA-Tyr3-octreotide PET in neuroendocrine tumors: comparison with somatostatin receptor scintigraphy and CT. J Nucl Med 2007;48(4):508–18.

8. Ambrosini V, Campana D, Tomassetti P, et al. 68Ga-labelled SSTRTs for diagnosis of gastroentero-pancreatic NET. Eur J Nucl Med Mol Imaging 2012; 39(Suppl 1):S52–60.

9. Virgolini I, Ambrosini V, Bomanji JB, et al. Procedure guidelines for PET/CT tumour imaging with 68Ga-DOTA-conjugated SSTRTs: 68Ga-DOTA-TOC, 68Ga-DOTA-NOC, 68Ga-DOTA-TATE. Eur J Nucl Med Mol Imaging 2010;37(10):2004–10.

10. Poeppel TD, Binse I, Petersenn S, et al. 68Ga-DOTATOC versus 68Ga-DOTATATE PET/CT in functional imaging of neuroendocrine tumors. J Nucl Med 2011;52(12):1864–70.

11. Kabasakal L, Demirci E, Ocak M, et al. Comparison of 68Ga-DOTATATE and 68Ga-DOTANOC PET/CT imaging in the same patient group with neuroendocrine tumours. Eur J Nucl Med Mol Imaging 2012; 39(8):1271–7.

12. Srirajaskanthan R, Kayani I, Quigley AM, et al. The role of 68Ga-DOTATATE PET in patients with neuroendocrine tumors and negative or equivocal findings on 111In-DTPA-octreotide scintigraphy. J Nucl Med 2010;51(6):875–82.

13. Ambrosini V, Campana D, Bodei L, et al. 68Ga-DOTANOC PET/CT clinical impact in patients with neuroendocrine tumors. J Nucl Med 2010;51(5): 669–73.

14. Campana D, Ambrosini V, Pezzilli R, et al. Standardized uptake values of (68)Ga-DOTANOC PET: a promising prognostic tool in neuroendocrine tumors. J Nucl Med 2010;51(3):353–9.

15. Kaemmerer D, Peter L, Lupp A, et al. Molecular imaging with 68Ga-SSTR PET/CT and correlation to immunohistochemistry of somatostatin receptors in neuroendocrine tumours. Eur J Nucl Med Mol Imaging 2011;38(9):1659–68.

16. Prasad V, Ambrosini V, Hommann M, et al. Detection of unknown primary neuroendocrine tumours (CUP-NET) using (68)Ga-DOTA-NOC receptor PET/CT. Eur J Nucl Med Mol Imaging 2010;37(1):67–77.

17. Ambrosini V, Tomassetti P, Castellucci P, et al. Comparison between 68Ga-DOTA-NOC and 18F-DOPA PET for the detection of gastro-entero-pancreatic and lung neuroendocrine tumours. Eur J Nucl Med Mol Imaging 2008;35(8):1431–8.

18. Haug A, Auernhammer CJ, Wängler B, et al. Intraindividual comparison of 68Ga-DOTA-TATE and 18F-DOPA PET in patients with well-differentiated metastatic neuroendocrine tumours. Eur J Nucl Med Mol Imaging 2009;36(5):765–70.

19. Koopmans KP, Neels ON, Kema IP, et al. Molecular imaging in neuroendocrine tumors: molecular uptake mechanisms and clinical results. Crit Rev Oncol Hematol 2009;71(3):199–213.

20. Velikyan I, Beyer GJ, Långström B. Microwave-supported preparation of 68Ga bioconjugates with high specific radioactivity. Bioconjug Chem 2004; 15:554–60.

21. Meyer GJ, Maecke H, Schuhmacher J, et al. 68Ga-labelled DOTA-derivatised peptide ligands. Eur J Nucl Med Mol Imaging 2004;31:1097–104.

22. Zhernosekov KP, Filosofov DV, Baum RP, et al. Processing of generator-produced 68Ga for medical application. J Nucl Med 2007;48:1741–8.

23. Breeman WA, de Jong M, de Blois E, et al. Radiolabelling DOTA-SSTRTs with 68Ga. Eur J Nucl Med Mol Imaging 2005;32:478–85.

24. Decristoforo C, Knopp R, von Guggenberg E, et al. A fully automated synthesis for the preparation of 68Ga-labelled SSTRTs. Nucl Med Commun 2007; 28:870–5.

25. Mayerhoefer ME, Schuetz M, Magnaldi S, et al. Are contrast media required for (68)Ga-DOTA-TOC PET/CT in patients with neuroendocrine tumours of the abdomen? Eur Radiol 2012;22(4): 938–46.

26. Castellucci P, Pou Ucha J, Fuccio C, et al. Incidence of increased 68Ga-DOTANOC uptake in the pancreatic head in a large series of extrapancreatic NET patients studied with sequential PET/CT. J Nucl Med 2011;52(6):886–90.

Proliferation Imaging with ^{18}F-Fluorothymidine PET/Computed Tomography
Physiologic Uptake, Variants, and Pitfalls

Ken Herrmann, MD*, Andreas K. Buck, MD

KEYWORDS

- PET/CT • ^{18}F-fluorothymidine • Proliferation • Cancer • Pitfalls • Physiologic variation

KEY POINTS

- For noninvasive in vivo imaging of proliferation, 3′-deoxy-3′-[^{18}F]fluorothymidine (^{18}F-FLT) PET combined with computed tomography (PET/CT) remains a promising tool, owing its correlation with proliferation indexes in many tumor entities.
- Future clinical applications will focus on monitoring response to cancer therapy, whereas tumor detection will be limited to organs with high physiologic [^{18}F]fluorodeoxyglucose uptake.
- Use and interpretation of ^{18}F-FLT requires knowledge of the physiologic tracer distribution and how it will be affected by anticancer treatment.
- Further studies are needed to determine the optimal timing of ^{18}F-FLT PET/CT imaging in the course of cancer therapies or at therapy conclusion.

INTRODUCTION

Diagnosis and treatment of cancer remains one of the biggest challenges in modern health care, and also plays a significant economic role. Reported direct cancer care costs in the United States for 2010 were an estimated $125 billion and are expected to increase to $173 billion in 2020.[1] These enormous expenditures are partly driven by the introduction of new cancer treatments but result in only modest survival improvement in most cancers,[2] underlining the need for ways to diagnose cancer early and to monitor response to treatment.[3]

Introduction of the noninvasive medical imaging technique [^{18}F]fluorodeoxyglucose (^{18}F-FDG) PET combined with computed tomography (PET/CT), together with the emergence of commercial distribution networks for ^{18}F-FDG and broadened coverage by the Centers of Medicare and Medicaid Services based on an extensive literature review,[4] changed the landscape of cancer imaging.[5] Despite the introduction of new tracers,[6] ^{18}F-FDG still accounts for most of the more than 2 million clinical PET/CT studies per year in the United States.

Retention of ^{18}F-FDG in the tumor reflects cellular growth and proliferation only in part. Moreover, ^{18}F-FDG uptake has also been reported to be associated with false-positive findings resulting from unspecific tracer uptake in inflammatory processes.[7,8] Therefore, to increase specificity for malignant lesions, other tracers that complement the information provided by ^{18}F-FDG are required and are gaining the attention of the scientific community.

Promising cellular processes for cancer imaging compiled in the article "The Hallmarks of Cancer," comprising angiogenesis, tumor invasion and metastases, apoptosis, inflammation, unstable DNA, and proliferation, were initially published in 2000 and recently updated.[9,10] As many anticancer

Department of Nuclear Medicine, Universitätsklinikum Würzburg, Oberdürrbacher Str. 6, Würzburg 97080, Germany
* Corresponding author.
E-mail address: kherrmann@mednet.ucla.edu

PET Clin 9 (2014) 331–338
http://dx.doi.org/10.1016/j.cpet.2014.03.005

drugs have been designed to inhibit cell proliferation and/or to induce apoptosis, in vivo assessment of proliferation seems a promising tool for imaging cancer and assessing response to treatment, potentially overcoming the limitations associated with ^{18}F-FDG PET imaging. Furthermore, imaging of proliferation potentially allows not only better differentiation between benign and malignant processes but also noninvasive grading and, hence, estimation of tumor aggressiveness.[11–14]

Noninvasive assessment of tumor growth and DNA synthesis might be appropriate for assessing proliferative activity in malignant tumors. Thus far several DNA precursors have been investigated, including [^{11}C]thymidine, which represents the native pyrimidine analogue used for DNA synthesis in vivo.[15] Because of the short half-life of ^{11}C and rapid degradation of [^{11}C]thymidine, this tracer was considered less suitable for clinical use. Recently, the thymidine analogue 3'-deoxy-3'-[^{18}F]fluorothymidine (^{18}F-FLT) was suggested for noninvasive assessment of proliferation and more specific tumor imaging.[16] The effort to synthesize ^{18}F-FLT is similar to that of the standard radiotracer ^{18}F-FDG.[17] ^{18}F-FLT, which is derived from the cytostatic drug azidothymidine (AZT), has been reported to be stable in vitro and to accumulate in proliferating tissues and malignant tumors.[16] Thymidine kinase 1 was identified as key enzyme responsible for the intracellular trapping of ^{18}F-FLT.[18,19] Recently, a significant correlation of tumor proliferation and ^{18}F-FLT uptake in various malignant tumors has been described, including breast cancer,[20] colorectal cancer,[21] lung cancer,[22] gliomas,[13,23] sarcomas,[11] and lymphomas.[24]

APPLICATIONS OF ^{18}F-FLT IN THE CLINIC

^{18}F-FLT PET has been widely investigated in the oncologic setting comprising tumor detection, staging, restaging, and assessment of response to treatment.[25]

First studies focused on tumor detection in lung tumors,[26] sarcoma,[14] breast cancer,[27] colorectal cancer,[21] esophageal cancer,[28] and melanoma,[29] often comparing ^{18}F-FLT PET with the more established PET tracer ^{18}F-FDG. More recently, ^{18}F-FLT PET has been primarily used for assessing response to anticancer treatment, including cytotoxic drugs, targeted agents, radiotherapy, and combination treatment.[25] The main rationale for expanding the use of ^{18}F-FLT PET in treatment monitoring is the rapid decline of the ^{18}F-FLT uptake observed as soon as a few days after the initiation of treatment, in addition to the antiproliferative origin of numerous newly developed drugs. Use of ^{18}F-FLT PET for response monitoring has been reported, among other tumor subtypes, for hematologic malignancies,[30,31] sarcomas,[32,33] breast cancer,[34,35] glioma,[36,37] gastrointestinal tumors,[38–40] genitourinary cancers,[41] head and neck cancers,[42,43] lung cancers,[44,45] and skin cancers[46,47] (for a review, see Ref.[25]).

HEAD AND NECK

As ^{18}F-FLT does not cross the intact blood-brain barrier (BBB), the physiologic brain uptake is low, especially in comparison with ^{18}F-FDG (**Fig. 1**). Breakdown of the BBB, however, can cause significant ^{18}F-FLT retention without present cell proliferation. Nevertheless, ^{18}F-FLT has been reported to be useful for the detection[13,23] and treatment monitoring of gliomas,[36,37] although a differentiation between high-grade and low-grade tumors was not possible.

The physiologic ^{18}F-FLT uptake in the neck region is low, and ^{18}F-FLT PET was therefore believed to discriminate between inflammatory and neoplastic lymph node involvement. However, Troost and colleagues[48] reported false-positive ^{18}F-FLT uptake in 6 of 9 patients with visually positive lymph nodes. Histopathologic analysis and immunostaining identified the germinal centers of

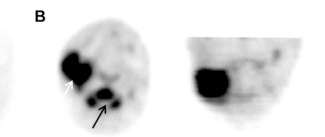

Fig. 1. (A) Transaxial and coronal view of ^{18}F-FLT PET of the head, indicating the physiologic low brain ^{18}F-FLT uptake. (B) Corresponding transaxial and coronal ^{18}F-FLT PET images of a patient with retromandibular lymphoma (*white arrow*) and physiologic tracer uptake in the cervical vertebrae (*black arrow*).

B lymphocytes to be the origin of the increased inflammatory ^{18}F-FLT uptake.

Further areas of physiologic ^{18}F-FLT uptake in the head and neck region include proliferating bone marrow present in the cervical spine and, to a lesser extent, the skull (see **Fig. 1**). The high physiologic ^{18}F-FLT uptake throughout the proliferating bone marrow reduces the sensitivity regarding bone marrow infiltration and primary and secondary bone lesions.[49,50] Nevertheless, in patients with aggressive non-Hodgkin lymphoma (NHL), even osseous lesions were detectable because focal ^{18}F-FLT uptake was greater than in the surrounding bone marrow.[51] The high physiologic ^{18}F-FLT uptake in proliferating bone marrow was also successfully used to visualize the viable bone marrow compartment in patients with aplastic anemia, and to identify organs with ongoing extraosseous hematopoiesis.[52]

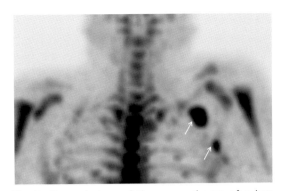

Fig. 2. Coronal view of the upper thorax of a lymphoma patient undergoing ^{18}F-FLT PET for staging. The lung itself shows only very low uptake, whereas physiologic ^{18}F-FLT uptake can be seen in the proliferating bone marrow of the cervical and thoracic vertebrae, the rib cage, and both humeri. Despite the physiologic ^{18}F-FLT uptake, the lymphoma manifestations are visually easily detectable (*white arrows*).

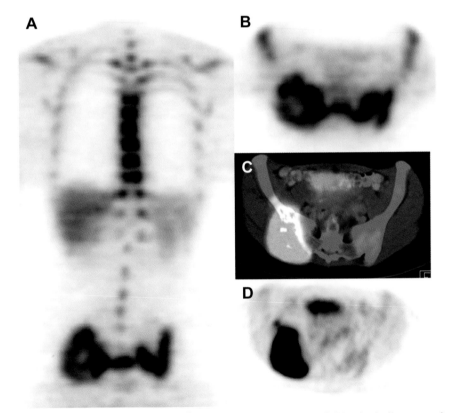

Fig. 3. Coronal (*A*) and transaxial (*B*) views of ^{18}F-FLT PET for a patient with histologically proven lymphoma in sacrum and right iliac bone. The images indicate the high physiologic ^{18}F-FLT uptake throughout the proliferating bone marrow, the comparable low physiologic ^{18}F-FLT uptake of liver and spleen in addition to the lung. Despite the physiologic ^{18}F-FLT uptake in the proliferating bone marrow, the lymphoma manifestations are easily visually depicted. For comparison, the corresponding transaxial-view ^{18}F-FDG PET/CT, (*C*) fused ^{18}F-FDG PET/CT, and (*D*) ^{18}F-FDG PET images are shown. (*Adapted from* Herrmann K, Buck AK, Schuster T, et al. Predictive value of initial ^{18}F-FLT uptake in patients with aggressive non-Hodgkin lymphoma receiving R-CHOP treatment. J Nucl Med 2011;52:690–6; with permission.)

THORAX

Physiologic lung parenchyma shows only very low ^{18}F-FLT uptake, and therefore permits the proposal that any kind of increased pulmonary ^{18}F-FLT uptake has to be rated as highly suspicious for a malignant tumor (**Fig. 2**). Increased physiologic ^{18}F-FLT uptake might be seen in the heart region because of accumulation of FLT in the blood pool and muscle tissue of the left ventricular cavity, potentially obscuring lung and breast lesions.[53] However, the blood pool activity in the heart is washed out quickly, as shown in time-activity curves, and allows good visualization of the thorax after around 45 minutes[53] with a reported mean standardized uptake value (SUV$_{mean}$) of 2.2 in the heart at 60 minutes postinjection (compared with 12.2 in the liver and 16.0 in the vertebrae). An approach to overcome this limitation was the development of a classification algorithm isolating cancerous tissue from healthy organs.[53] Application of this filter led to a reduction of 80% of the liver and heart signal, whereas the corresponding signal in primary breast tumors and metastases was mainly retained.

Further physiologic ^{18}F-FLT uptake in the thoracic region can be found in the rib cage and the thoracic vertebrae, owing to the presence of the proliferation bone marrow. Implications regarding the bone marrow compartment are more extensively discussed in the section on the head and neck.

ABDOMEN

The abdomen contains several organs with increased physiologic ^{18}F-FLT uptake, including the liver and, to a lesser extent, the intestines, in addition to the lower part of the rib cage and the corresponding thoracic and lumbar vertebrae (**Fig. 3**).

Whereas in rabbits, dogs, and mice the weakest hepatic ^{18}F-FLT uptake has been observed, a relatively high hepatic accumulation of ^{18}F-FLT can be seen in humans (**Fig. 4**). ^{18}F-FLT undergoes extensive glucuronidation in the human liver, resulting in approximately 25% of the plasma activity being present as ^{18}F-FLT–glucuronide at 60 minutes after injection.[54–56] The reported SUV$_{mean}$ at 60 minutes postinjection was 12.2, derived from 29

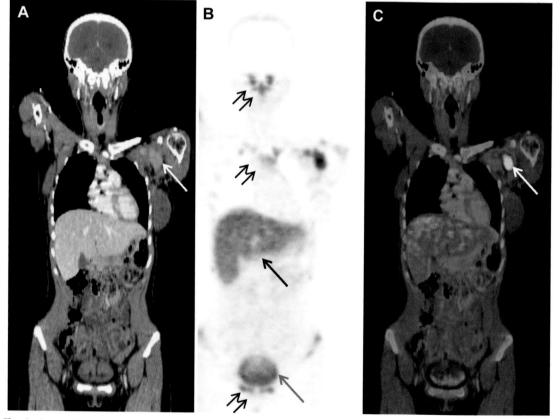

Fig. 4. Coronal views of CT (*A*), PET (*B*), and fused PET/CT (*C*) of a patient with lymphoma of the left axilla (*white arrows*) undergoing ^{18}F-FLT PET/CT. Physiologic ^{18}F-FLT uptake is seen in the liver (*black arrow*), in the bladder (*red arrow*), and in the proliferating bone marrow scans (*black double arrows*).

scans in 15 patients with breast cancer.[53] Despite this high physiologic uptake in the liver, 13 of 18 patients with suspected hepatocellular carcinoma showed higher than surrounding liver activity and were visually detectable as hot lesions, resulting in sensitivity of 72%.[57] Attempts to reduce the physiologic liver uptake of ^{18}F-FLT by use of probenecid, previously shown to reduce the glucuronidation of AZT in patients being treated for human immunodeficiency virus,[58] failed in a pilot evaluation.[55]

Physiologic uptake in the gastrointestinal mucosa is somewhat expected, as the mucosa cells are known to undergo rapid proliferation. ^{18}F-FLT uptake in normal gastric wall was recently measured in 25 patients with a mean maximum SUV (SUV_{max}) of 1.8 (range 1.0–2.6).[59] Corresponding mean SUV_{max} of the gastric tumor lesion was 7.3 (range 2.0–25.3). A cutoff value of $SUV_{max} = 2.6$ resulted in no false-positive findings and a corresponding sensitivity of 94.7% for detection of gastric carcinoma. The finding that physiologic gastrointestinal ^{18}F-FLT uptake does not include the detection of gastric cancer was confirmed by multiple groups.[60,61]

As discussed earlier in the section on the head and neck, physiologic ^{18}F-FLT uptake is perceived throughout the proliferating bone marrow in the lower rib cage as well as in the lumbar spine.

PELVIS AND GENITOURINARY SYSTEM

^{18}F-FLT is excreted by the kidneys mainly in its nonmetabolized form, but also as ^{18}F-FLT-glucuronide after being metabolized in the liver.[54] At 60 minutes postinjection, there is only low nonspecific ^{18}F-FLT retention in the kidneys and the genitourinary system. Sometimes seen, and always important to take into account, are urinary contaminations.

More relevant for the visual interpretation is the high physiologic ^{18}F-FLT uptake in the proliferating bone marrow often seen throughout the pelvic bones and the lumbar vertebrae, as more extensively discussed in the section on the head and neck (**Fig. 5**).

Other pelvic organs, such as the uterus and ovaries, prostate, and seminal vesicles, do not show any significant physiologic ^{18}F-FLT uptake.

EFFECTS OF AGING AND TREATMENT
Aging

The extent of proliferating bone marrow as the primary source of physiologic ^{18}F-FLT uptake in humans changes from the newborn to the elderly.

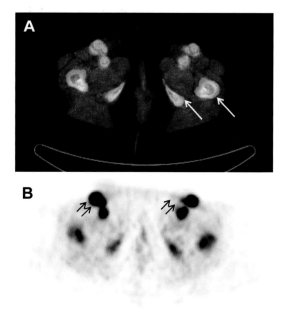

Fig. 5. Transaxial views of fused PET/CT (*A*) and PET (*B*) of the lower pelvis in a patient with mantle-cell lymphoma undergoing staging before therapy. In addition to the pathologic ^{18}F-FLT uptake seen in the inguinal lymph nodes (*black double arrows*), physiologic ^{18}F-FLT uptake can be identified in the proliferating bone marrow (*white arrows*).

With the exception of bone marrow, physiologic ^{18}F-FLT uptake is not subject to age-dependent alterations.

Treatment-Induced Effects

^{18}F-FLT PET has been widely used in a numerous studies and tumor entities for assessing the response to treatment (for review, see Refs.[25,62]). Response to chemotherapy is expected to result in a reduced ^{18}F-FLT uptake, as previously reported, for example, in malignant lymphomas (**Fig. 6**).[30] In patients undergoing chemoradiotherapy, increased ^{18}F-FLT uptake (so-called flare) 20 hours after irradiation of 2 Gy was reported in a patient with a non–small cell lung cancer.[63] Of note, treatment of aggressive NHL with rituximab alone, a chimeric monoclonal antibody directed against the antigen CD20, did not result in decreased ^{18}F-FLT uptake, and in some patients even increased ^{18}F-FLT uptake was reported.[30] Radiation and chemoradiotherapy also potentially affects the proliferating bone marrow compartment, explaining therapy-induced reduction of ^{18}F-FLT uptake. Photopenic regions are often seen after radiation therapy, for example in the spine. The antiproliferative effect of chemotherapy was also seen in aggressive NHL patients, with significantly decreased ^{18}F-FLT uptake 2 days after CHOP

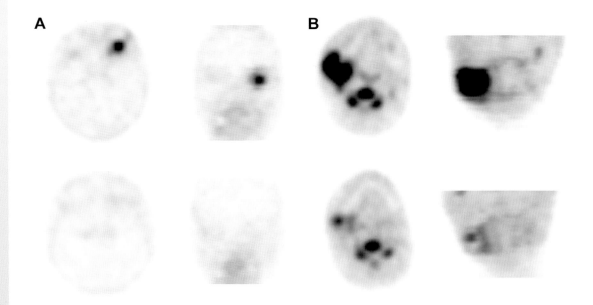

Fig. 6. Transaxial and coronal views of pretreatment ^{18}F-FLT PET scans (*upper panel*) of 2 lymphoma patients with retro-orbital (*A*) and retromandibular lymphoma (*B*). Corresponding early treatment response scans (*lower panel*) show no remaining visual uptake (*A*) and only low residual uptake (*B*) as soon as 5 days after start of chemotherapy. (*Adapted from* Herrmann K, Buck AK, Schuster T, et al. Predictive value of initial ^{18}F-FLT uptake in patients with aggressive non-Hodgkin lymphoma receiving R-CHOP treatment. J Nucl Med 2011;52:690–6; with permission.)

(cyclophosphamide/adriamycin/vincristine/prednisone) treatment, and almost again normalized ^{18}F-FLT uptake at day +7 and day +42.[30] In patients with renal cell carcinoma undergoing treatment with sunitinib, increased ^{18}F-FLT uptake was seen after withdrawal of sunitinib, a phenomenon called "withdrawal flare" by the investigators.[41]

SUMMARY

For noninvasive in vivo imaging of proliferation, ^{18}F-FLT PET/CT remains a promising tool, owing to its correlation with proliferation indexes in many tumor entities. Future clinical applications will focus on monitoring response to cancer therapy, whereas tumor detection will be limited to organs with high physiologic ^{18}F-FDG uptake. Use and interpretation of ^{18}F-FLT requires knowledge of the physiologic tracer distribution and how it will be affected by anticancer treatment. Further studies are needed to determine the optimal timing of ^{18}F-FLT PET/CT imaging in the course of cancer therapies or at the conclusion of therapy.

REFERENCES

1. Mariotto AB, Yabroff KR, Shao Y, et al. Projections of the cost of cancer care in the United States: 2010-2020. J Natl Cancer Inst 2011;103(2):117–28.

2. Parkin DM, Bray F, Ferlay J, et al. Global cancer statistics, 2002. CA Cancer J Clin 2005;55(2):74–108.

3. Yang Y, Czernin J. Contribution of imaging to cancer care costs. J Nucl Med 2011;52(Suppl 2):86S–92S.

4. Gambhir SS, Czernin J, Schwimmer J, et al. A tabulated summary of the FDG PET literature. J Nucl Med 2001;42(Suppl 5):1S–93S.

5. Czernin J, Allen-Auerbach M, Nathanson D, et al. PET/CT in oncology: current status and perspectives. Curr Radiol Rep 2013;1(3):177–90.

6. Kumar R, Dhanpathi H, Basu S, et al. Oncologic PET tracers beyond [(18)F]FDG and the novel quantitative approaches in PET imaging. Q J Nucl Med Mol Imaging 2008;52(1):50–65.

7. Kubota R, Kubota K, Yamada S, et al. Microautoradiographic study for the differentiation of intratumoral macrophages, granulation tissues and cancer cells by the dynamics of fluorine-18-fluorodeoxyglucose uptake. J Nucl Med 1994; 35(1):104–12.

8. Shreve PD, Anzai Y, Wahl RL. Pitfalls in oncologic diagnosis with FDG PET imaging: physiologic and benign variants. Radiographics 1999;19(1):61–77 [quiz: 150–1].

9. Hanahan D, Weinberg RA. The hallmarks of cancer. Cell 2000;100(1):57–70.

10. Hanahan D, Weinberg RA. Hallmarks of cancer: the next generation. Cell 2011;144(5):646–74.

11. Buck AK, Herrmann K, Buschenfelde CM, et al. Imaging bone and soft tissue tumors with the proliferation marker ^{18}F]fluorodeoxythymidine. Clin Cancer Res 2008;14(10):2970–7.

12. Buck AK, Kratochwil C, Glatting G, et al. Early assessment of therapy response in malignant lymphoma with the thymidine analogue ^{18}F-FLT. Eur J Nucl Med Mol Imaging 2007;34(11):1775–82.

13. Choi SJ, Kim JS, Kim JH, et al. [18]F]3'-deoxy-3'-fluorothymidine PET for the diagnosis and grading of brain tumors. Eur J Nucl Med Mol Imaging 2005; 32(6):653–9.

14. Cobben DC, Elsinga PH, Suurmeijer AJ, et al. Detection and grading of soft tissue sarcomas of the extremities with (18)F-3'-fluoro-3'-deoxy-L-thymidine. Clin Cancer Res 2004;10(5):1685–90.

15. Wells P, Gunn RN, Alison M, et al. Assessment of proliferation in vivo using 2-[C-11]thymidine positron emission tomography in advanced intra-abdominal malignancies. Cancer Res 2002;62(20):5698–702.

16. Shields AF, Grierson JR, Dohmen BM, et al. Imaging proliferation in vivo with ^{18}F-FLT and positron emission tomography. Nat Med 1998;4(11):1334–6.

17. Machulla HJ, Blocher A, Kuntzsch M, et al. Simplified labeling approach for synthesizing 3'-Deoxy-3'-^{18}F]fluorothymidine (^{18}F-FLT). J Radioanal Nucl Chem 2000;243(3):843–6.

18. Barthel H, Perumal M, Latigo J, et al. The uptake of 3'-deoxy-3'-^{18}F]fluorothymidine into L5178Y tumours in vivo is dependent on thymidine kinase 1 protein levels. Eur J Nucl Med Mol Imaging 2005; 32(3):257–63.

19. Rasey JS, Grierson JR, Wiens LW, et al. Validation of FLT uptake as a measure of thymidine kinase-1 activity in A549 carcinoma cells. J Nucl Med 2002;43(9):1210–7.

20. Kenny LM, Vigushin DM, Al-Nahhas A, et al. Quantification of cellular proliferation in tumor and normal tissues of patients with breast cancer by ^{18}F]fluorothymidine-positron emission tomography imaging: evaluation of analytical methods. Cancer Res 2005;65(21):10104–12.

21. Francis DL, Visvikis D, Costa DC, et al. Potential impact of ^{18}F]3'-deoxy-3'-fluorothymidine versus ^{18}F]fluoro-2-deoxy-D-glucose in positron emission tomography for colorectal cancer. Eur J Nucl Med Mol Imaging 2003;30(7):988–94.

22. Buck AK, Schirrmeister H, Hetzel M, et al. 3-deoxy-3-[(18)F]fluorothymidine-positron emission tomography for noninvasive assessment of proliferation in pulmonary nodules. Cancer Res 2002;62(12):3331–4.

23. Chen W, Cloughesy T, Kamdar N, et al. Imaging proliferation in brain tumors with ^{18}F-FLT PET: comparison with ^{18}F-FDG. J Nucl Med 2005; 46(6):945–52.

24. Wagner M, Seitz U, Buck A, et al. 3'-^{18}F]fluoro-3'-deoxythymidine (^{18}F-FLT) as positron emission tomography tracer for imaging proliferation in a murine B-Cell lymphoma model and in the human disease. Cancer Res 2003;63(10):2681–7.

25. Tehrani OS, Shields AF. PET imaging of proliferation with pyrimidines. J Nucl Med 2013;54(6):903–12.

26. Buck AK, Halter G, Schirrmeister H, et al. Imaging proliferation in lung tumors with PET: ^{18}F-FLT versus ^{18}F-FDG. J Nucl Med 2003;44(9):1426–31.

27. Smyczek-Gargya B, Fersis N, Dittmann H, et al. PET with ^{18}F]fluorothymidine for imaging of primary breast cancer: a pilot study. Eur J Nucl Med Mol Imaging 2004;31(5):720–4.

28. van Westreenen HL, Westerterp M, Jager PL, et al. Synchronous primary neoplasms detected on ^{18}F-FDG PET in staging of patients with esophageal cancer. J Nucl Med 2005;46(8):1321–5.

29. Cobben DC, Jager PL, Elsinga PH, et al. 3'-^{18}F-fluoro-3'-deoxy-L-thymidine: a new tracer for staging metastatic melanoma? J Nucl Med 2003;44(12): 1927–32.

30. Herrmann K, Wieder HA, Buck AK, et al. Early response assessment using 3'-deoxy-3'-^{18}F]fluorothymidine-positron emission tomography in high-grade non-Hodgkin's lymphoma. Clin Cancer Res 2007;13(12):3552–8.

31. Lee H, Kim SK, Kim YI, et al. Early determination of prognosis by interim 3'-deoxy-3'-^{18}F-fluorothymidine PET in patients with non-Hodgkin lymphoma. J Nucl Med 2014;55(2):216–22.

32. Been LB, Suurmeijer AJ, Elsinga PH, et al. ^{18}F-Fluorodeoxythymidine PET for evaluating the response to hyperthermic isolated limb perfusion for locally advanced soft-tissue sarcomas. J Nucl Med 2007;48(3):367–72.

33. Benz MR, Czernin J, Allen-Auerbach MS, et al. 3'-deoxy-3'-^{18}F]fluorothymidine positron emission tomography for response assessment in soft tissue sarcoma: a pilot study to correlate imaging findings with tissue thymidine kinase 1 and Ki-67 activity and histopathologic response. Cancer 2012; 118(12):3135–44.

34. Contractor KB, Kenny LM, Stebbing J, et al. [18]F]-3'Deoxy-3'-fluorothymidine positron emission tomography and breast cancer response to docetaxel. Clin Cancer Res 2011;17(24):7664–72.

35. Pio BS, Park CK, Pietras R, et al. Usefulness of 3'-[F-18]fluoro-3'-deoxythymidine with positron emission tomography in predicting breast cancer response to therapy. Mol Imaging Biol 2006;8(1):36–42.

36. Harris RJ, Cloughesy TF, Pope WB, et al. ^{18}F-FDOPA and ^{18}F-FLT positron emission tomography parametric response maps predict response in recurrent malignant gliomas treated with bevacizumab. Neuro Oncol 2012;14(8):1079–89.

37. Schwarzenberg J, Czernin J, Cloughesy TF, et al. 3'-deoxy-3'-^{18}F-fluorothymidine PET and MRI for early survival predictions in patients with recurrent

malignant glioma treated with bevacizumab. J Nucl Med 2012;53(1):29–36.

38. Ott K, Herrmann K, Schuster T, et al. Molecular imaging of proliferation and glucose utilization: utility for monitoring response and prognosis after neoadjuvant therapy in locally advanced gastric cancer. Ann Surg Oncol 2011;18(12):3316–23.

39. Wieder HA, Geinitz H, Rosenberg R, et al. PET imaging with [18F]3'-deoxy-3'-fluorothymidine for prediction of response to neoadjuvant treatment in patients with rectal cancer. Eur J Nucl Med Mol Imaging 2007;34(6):878–83.

40. Yue J, Chen L, Cabrera AR, et al. Measuring tumor cell proliferation with 18F-FLT PET during radiotherapy of esophageal squamous cell carcinoma: a pilot clinical study. J Nucl Med 2010;51(4):528–34.

41. Liu G, Jeraj R, Vanderhoek M, et al. Pharmacodynamic study using FLT PET/CT in patients with renal cell cancer and other solid malignancies treated with sunitinib malate. Clin Cancer Res 2011;17(24):7634–44.

42. Kishino T, Hoshikawa H, Nishiyama Y, et al. Usefulness of 3'-deoxy-3'-18F-fluorothymidine PET for predicting early response to chemoradiotherapy in head and neck cancer. J Nucl Med 2012;53(10):1521–7.

43. Troost EG, Bussink J, Hoffmann AL, et al. 18F-FLT PET/CT for early response monitoring and dose escalation in oropharyngeal tumors. J Nucl Med 2010;51(6):866–74.

44. Trigonis I, Koh PK, Taylor B, et al. Early reduction in tumour [18F]fluorothymidine (FLT) uptake in patients with non-small cell lung cancer (NSCLC) treated with radiotherapy alone. Eur J Nucl Med Mol Imaging 2014;41(4):682–93.

45. Zander T, Scheffler M, Nogova L, et al. Evaluation of the accuracy of FDG-/FLT-PET for early prediction of non-progression in patients with advanced non-small cell lung cancer (NSCLC) treated with erlotinib. J Clin Oncol 2009;27(15). Available at: http://meeting.ascopubs.org/cgi/content/abstract/27/15S/e19054.

46. Aarntzen EH, Srinivas M, De Wilt JH, et al. Early identification of antigen-specific immune responses in vivo by [18F]-labeled 3'-fluoro-3'-deoxy-thymidine (18F-FLT) PET imaging. Proc Natl Acad Sci U S A 2011;108(45):18396–9.

47. Ribas A, Benz MR, Allen-Auerbach MS, et al. Imaging of CTLA4 blockade-induced cell replication with 18F-FLT PET in patients with advanced melanoma treated with tremelimumab. J Nucl Med 2010;51(3):340–6.

48. Troost EG, Vogel WV, Merkx MA, et al. 18F-FLT PET does not discriminate between reactive and metastatic lymph nodes in primary head and neck cancer patients. J Nucl Med 2007;48(5):726–35.

49. Buck AK, Herrmann K, Shen C, et al. Molecular imaging of proliferation in vivo: positron emission tomography with [18F]fluorothymidine. Methods 2009;48(2):205–15.

50. Buck AK, Bommer M, Stilgenbauer S, et al. Molecular imaging of proliferation in malignant lymphoma. Cancer Res 2006;66(22):11055–61.

51. Herrmann K, Buck AK, Schuster T, et al. Predictive value of initial 18F-FLT uptake in patients with aggressive non-Hodgkin lymphoma receiving R-CHOP treatment. J Nucl Med 2011;52(5):690–6.

52. Agool A, Slart RH, Kluin PM, et al. 18F-FLT PET: a noninvasive diagnostic tool for visualization of the bone marrow compartment in patients with aplastic anemia: a pilot study. Clin Nucl Med 2011;36(4):286–9.

53. Gray KR, Contractor KB, Kenny LM, et al. Kinetic filtering of [(18)F]Fluorothymidine in positron emission tomography studies. Phys Med Biol 2010;55(3):695–709.

54. Muzi M, Mankoff DA, Grierson JR, et al. Kinetic modeling of 3'-deoxy-3'-fluorothymidine in somatic tumors: mathematical studies. J Nucl Med 2005;46(2):371–80.

55. Shields AF, Briston DA, Chandupatla S, et al. A simplified analysis of [18F]3'-deoxy-3'-fluorothymidine metabolism and retention. Eur J Nucl Med Mol Imaging 2005;32(11):1269–75.

56. Visvikis D, Francis D, Mulligan R, et al. Comparison of methodologies for the in vivo assessment of 18FLT utilisation in colorectal cancer. Eur J Nucl Med Mol Imaging 2004;31(2):169–78.

57. Eckel F, Herrmann K, Schmidt S, et al. Imaging of proliferation in hepatocellular carcinoma with the in vivo marker 18F-fluorothymidine. J Nucl Med 2009;50(9):1441–7.

58. Hedaya MA, Elmquist WF, Sawchuk RJ. Probenecid inhibits the metabolic and renal clearances of zidovudine (AZT) in human volunteers. Pharm Res 1990;7(4):411–7.

59. Malkowski B, Staniuk T, Srutek E, et al. 18F-FLT PET/CT in patients with gastric carcinoma. Gastroenterol Res Pract 2013;2013:696423.

60. Kameyama R, Yamamoto Y, Izuishi K, et al. Detection of gastric cancer using 18F-FLT PET: comparison with 18F-FDG PET. Eur J Nucl Med Mol Imaging 2009;36(3):382–8.

61. Herrmann K, Ott K, Buck AK, et al. Imaging gastric cancer with PET and the radiotracers 18F-FLT and 18F-FDG: a comparative analysis. J Nucl Med 2007;48(12):1945–50.

62. Bading JR, Shields AF. Imaging of cell proliferation: status and prospects. J Nucl Med 2008;49(Suppl 2):64S–80S.

63. Everitt S, Hicks RJ, Ball D, et al. Imaging cellular proliferation during chemo-radiotherapy: a pilot study of serial 18F-FLT positron emission tomography/computed tomography imaging for non-small-cell lung cancer. Int J Radiat Oncol Biol Phys 2009;75(4):1098–104.

11C-Acetate PET/CT Imaging
Physiologic Uptake, Variants, and Pitfalls

Georgios Karanikas, MD[a],*,
Mohsen Beheshti, MD, FASNC, FEBNM[b]

KEYWORDS

- PET-CT • Acetate • Pitfalls • Physiologic distribution

KEY POINTS

- ^{11}C-acetate is a biomarker for cell membrane lipid synthesis and may increase in various malignancies.
- Enhanced uptake is observed in salivary glands, tonsils, meningeal tuberculoma, meningiomas, macroadenomas of pituitary gland, and benign thyroid nodes.
- Reactive lymphadenopathy in mediastinum and hilum shows mild to moderate ^{11}C-acetate accumulation.
- Pancreas, spleen, and liver show an increased uptake of ^{11}C-acetate; however, pancreatitis is related with reduced tracer accumulation.
- Proliferative or granulomatous cystitis may be present with enhanced ^{11}C-acetate tracer accumulation.

This article describes the physiologic distribution of ^{11}C-acetate and discusses regions that occasionally may present increased activity not related to tumor tissue or owing to other nononcologic findings. The short half-life of ^{11}C-acetate (20 min) warrants an onsite cyclotron. Hence, there are less data available comparing ^{18}F-labeled PET tracers.

[11]C-acetate PET has been used to measure myocardial oxygen consumption and to study prostate cancer (PCa), hepatocellular carcinoma (HCC), renal cell carcinoma (RCC), bladder carcinoma, and brain tumors.[1] There are also rare conditions that have been incidentally depicted by ^{11}C-acetate PET, such as thymoma,[2] cerebellopontine angle schwannoma,[3] angiomyolipoma of the kidney,[4] and encephalitis.[5] Assessment of multiple myeloma has also been studied by this tracer.[6]

Acetate is a molecule quickly picked up by cells and converted into acetyl-CoA by acetyl-CoA synthetase.[1] It is used to synthesize cholesterol and fatty acids, thus forming cell membrane (anabolic pathway), or is oxidized (catabolic pathway) in mitochondria by the tricarboxylic acid (TCA) cycle to CO_2 and H_2O, thus producing energy. The predominant pathway is strictly linked with the type of cell; in myocardial tissue, acetate is mainly metabolized to CO_2 via the TCA cycle,[7] whereas tumor cells overexpress the enzyme fatty acid synthetase, thus converting most of the acetate into fatty acids and incorporating them into intracellular phosphatidylcholine membrane microdomains that are important for tumor growth and metastasis.[8] For nuclear medicine purposes, acetate is labeled with ^{11}C, and the derived compound is called ^{11}C-acetate.

Conflict of Interest: The authors declare no conflict of interest.
[a] Division of Nuclear Medicine, PET-PET/CT, Department of Biomedical Imaging and Image-Guided Therapy, Medical University of Vienna, Waehringer Guertel 18-20, Vienna A-1090, Austria; [b] PET-CT Center LINZ, Department of Nuclear Medicine and Endocrinology, St. Vincent's Hospital, Seilerstaette 4, Linz A-4020, Austria
* Corresponding author.
E-mail address: georgios.karanikas@meduniwien.ac.at

Visual inspection of dynamic ^{11}C-acetate PET images demonstrated rapid accumulation of activity in the heart, kidneys, liver, pancreas, spleen, stomach, bowel, and bone marrow. The organs that received the highest absorbed doses were the pancreas (critical organ), bowel, kidneys, spleen, heart, and liver. ^{11}C-acetate has no measurable urinary excretion. No significant cerebral uptake was seen in the published study.[9]

As a routine protocol in the authors' centers, a fixed dose of about 740 MBq ^{11}C-acetate is administered intravenously through the cubital vein. Imaging of ^{11}C-acetate is similar to that performed with most PET radiopharmaceuticals, from the base of the skull to mid thighs or over the whole body, depending on the clinical indication. Acquisition starts 10 to 15 minutes postinjection. Whole-body protocol starts with a scout view, followed by the low-dose computed tomographic (CT) acquisition for attenuation correction and subsequent PET acquisition for 2 to 5 minutes for each of the 6 to 8 bed positions.

CENTRAL NERVOUS SYSTEM, HEAD, AND NECK

In the brain, acetate is preferentially metabolized by astrocytes, and labeled acetate has been used to assess glial metabolism and glial-neuronal interactions. Metabolic data derived from a small set of tumors revealed that glioblastoma and meningioma clearly can convert ^{14}C-acetate into acidic and amino acid metabolites, presumably through the oxidative pathway of the TCA cycle.[10] The uptake of ^{14}C-acetate was studied in 4 different tumor cell lines and a fibroblast cell line to investigate the metabolic pathway of ^{14}C-acetate in tumor cells. [14]C accumulation in each of the 4 tumor lines was higher than that in fibroblast cells, and this accumulation in tumor cells was shown to be caused by enhanced lipid synthesis.[11]

The rate of metabolism of acetate in the normal rat brain is lower and more homogeneous than the local rates of glucose use and slightly increases during physiologic stimulation. This advantage of radiolabeled acetate provides a stable low background and higher tumor to cortex ratio to delineate tumors. Increased uptake of ^{11}C-acetate was found in meningeal tuberculoma.[12] Inflammatory cells, especially macrophages, in the tuberculoma may be responsible for increased uptake of ^{11}C-acetate.

Meningiomas, usually benign, solitary tumor of the meninges, show high uptake of ^{11}C-acetate in contrast to low uptake in normal brain tissue.

[11]C-acetate was found to be useful for detecting meningiomas and evaluating the extent of meningiomas and potentially useful for monitoring tumor response to radiosurgery.[12] Macroadenomas of pituitary gland also show positive results on ^{11}C-acetate PET/CT acquisition.[13]

Benign thyroid nodes present enhanced activity of the tracer.[14] In all cases, a moderate to high uptake was observed in salivary glands and tonsils but no obvious retention of ^{11}C-acetate was observed in the normal nasopharynx (**Fig. 1**).[15] The other structures in the neck show no enhanced uptake of the tracer.[16]

THORAX

Lung parenchyma shows faint tracer accumulation, whereas the mediastinum presents a minor uptake. Diffuse increased uptake in the lungs correlates to lung parenchyma disease.[17] Reactive lymphadenopathy in mediastinum and hilum shows enhanced ^{11}C-acetate accumulation (symmetric pattern); these findings are usually

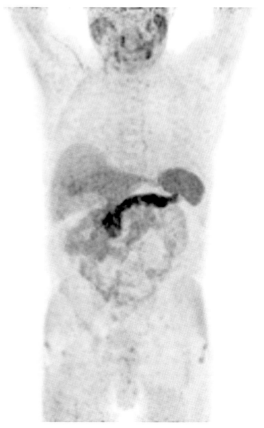

Fig. 1. Physiologic biodistribution of the tracer. The salivary glands and the upper abdominal parenchymatous organs such as liver, spleen, and pancreas show a major uptake of ^{11}C-acetate.

considered as reactive and/or inflammatory lymph nodes not related to primary tumor (**Fig. 2**). In addition, no tracer uptake is usually seen in the myocardium when performing routine oncologic protocol (ie, 20 minutes after intravenous injection).

Minor uptake was present in bone marrow, especially in dorsal vertebrae, whereas degenerative changes in the bones show an inhomogeneous moderate 11C-acetate uptake.

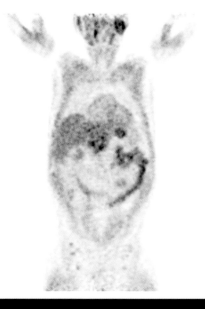

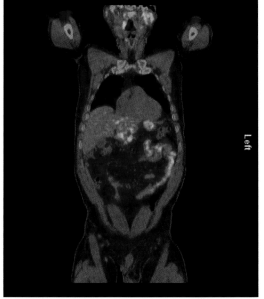

Fig. 2. Reactive inguinal lymphadenopathy shows enhanced 11C-acetate accumulation (symmetric hot spots).

ABDOMEN

The upper abdominal parenchymatous organs such as liver, spleen, and pancreas show an increased uptake of 11C-acetate. The highest uptake is found in pancreas, followed by spleen and then by liver (see **Fig. 1**). Uptake of 11C-acetate by pancreatic tissue is rapid, with the organ clearly visualized by 2 minutes. Tracer continues to accumulate in the pancreas relative to adjacent organs and background, such that by 10 minutes the pancreas is the most prominent organ in the imaging field. By 30 minutes postinjection, the pancreas remains well defined and is the only remaining conspicuous structure in the imaging field. The head, body, and tail of the pancreas are well delineated on images beyond 10 minutes because of the high target to background ratio. The pancreas to liver ratio 10 to 20 minutes postinjection ranged from 2.1 to 4.5, with a mean of 3.1, among the normal subjects studied. Pancreatic uptake of 11C-acetate was unaffected by pancreatic endocrine insufficiency but is absent in chronic pancreatitis complicated by exocrine insufficiency. Moderately reduced 11C-acetate uptake was observed in acute uncomplicated pancreatitis. The level of tracer accumulation was substantially reduced in phlegmatous masses complicating pancreatitis and in chronic mass forming pancreatitis. Adenocarcinoma of the pancreas likewise demonstrated no significant uptake of 11C-acetate. The high 11C-acetate tracer concentration within the pancreas is believed to be due to a high rate of lipid synthesis within pancreatic acinar cells.[18]

Focal nodular hyperplasia (FNH) and HCC are 11C-acetate-avid. However, they show different patterns of uptake and washout, especially with dual time imaging with delay acquisition.[19] In HCC, 11C-acetate activity in the delayed images is higher than in the early images, whereas in FNH, the 11C-acetate activity decreased in the delayed image when compared with early images.[19]

Previous studies reported that hemangioma; cholangiocarcinoma (pure primary adenocarcinoma of liver without HCC components); colon, breast, and lung cancers, and carcinoid tumors show no significant increased 11C-acetate uptake.[20] Increased tracer uptake may also be seen on the distal part of the esophagus, mainly due to the inflammatory process when performing gastroscopy.[21] In addition, low tracer uptake is seen in muscles, intestines, and renal parenchyma.

In normal subjects, the kidneys are clearly visualized with high target to background ratio relative to the soft tissues, liver, spleen, and pancreas by

60 seconds after tracer injection and remain the most prominent organ in the imaging field through 10 minutes. Because of the rapid clearance of renal tracer activity, pancreas tracer activity predominates after 10 minutes, and renal tracer activity rapidly approaches that of the liver, and eventually background. No urinary tracer activity appears at any time, and tracer distribution in the kidney has the configuration of the renal cortex. No urinary tracer activity was present in the intrarenal collecting system of any of the patients scanned, including those with renal disease. Even in patients with markedly reduced renal function due to chronic nephropathy with serum creatinine levels that exceeded 5 mg/dL, renal cortical tracer activity was readily identified. Like normal renal parenchyma, the 3 cases of RCC demonstrated high uptake of ^{11}C-acetate but differed markedly in the clearance of tissue tracer activity, which allows for clear differentiation of the neoplasm from normal tissue on image frames beyond 10 minutes of tracer administration. The loss of tracer activity from the tissue compartment is thus entirely due to flux of tracer back into the vascular compartment.[22] Renal complicated cysts without malignant tissue show negative ^{11}C-acetate findings.

PELVIS

The normal prostate shows usually only a minor uptake of the tracer. Focal inflammation of the prostate can cause increased focal tracer accumulation.[23] Dynamic prostate studies showed early high perfusion, with a maximum tracer uptake at about 5 minutes. Analysis of the individual time-activity curves revealed that the early uptake (standardized uptake value [SUV]-early), from 6 to 10 minutes, was, on average, similar to the late uptake, from 15 to 20 minutes. None of the early to late ratios was significantly different from unity. Subgroup analysis revealed that there was significantly different uptake in primary versus recurrent PCa, with SUV-late 3.84 versus 1.91 ($P<.001$), respectively. The range of SUV-late was 1.8 to 5.5 for primary cancer, 1.5 to 2.6 for recurrent cancer, and 3.2 to 3.5 for benign prostatic hyperplasia (BPH). The difference between BPH and recurrent cancer was significant ($P = .02$), but primary cancer could not be differentiated from BPH. A linear relationship between influx rate K and SUV-late was found for primary tumors ($r = 0.91$) but not for recurrent cancer ($r = -0.17$).[24] ^{11}C-acetate PET/CT demonstrates higher uptake in tumor foci than in normal prostate tissue.[25] Although ^{11}C-acetate PET/CT seems not to be an accurate diagnostic modality for the assessment of the primary glandular-confined PCa, it has the potential for guiding biopsy in individual clinically suspicious cases with negative biopsy results. In addition, because of its functional characteristics, ^{11}C-acetate seems to be useful for monitoring therapy, especially if anatomic structures were changed after surgery (**Fig. 3**). Prognostic value of ^{11}C-acetate PET/CT in PCa is still under debate and, to date, there are no sufficient data to draw a conclusion in this concern.[26]

In aerobic conditions, PC-3 and LNCaP cells exhibited an order of uptake preference as follows: choline > acetate > fluorodeoxyglucose. In hypoxic cells, the order is reversed, reflecting diverse biochemical responses to hypoxia. These findings may help to explain PET imaging findings of the diverse responses of these tracers in different stages and locations of PCa. Androgen deprivation markedly suppresses the uptake of all 3 tracers in LNCaP cells, which suggests the potential for underestimation of the disease state when PET imaging is performed after antiandrogen therapy.[27] There is no in vivo analysis for ^{11}C-acetate PET in this context.

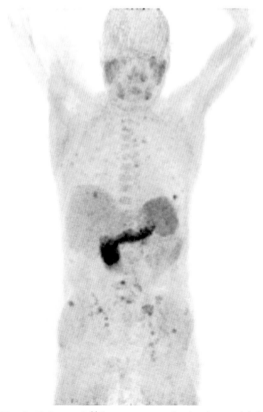

Fig. 3. Enhanced ^{11}C-acetate uptake in the multiple bone metastases in patient with recurrent prostate carcinoma.

Regularly, bowel shows a minor uptake, but rarely some patients present unusually high accumulation of acetate. In rare cases, patients had significant bladder and urethra uptake, whereas approximately half of the patients show significant uptake in the rectum. False-positive 11C-acetate uptake occurred because of proliferative or granulomatous cystitis.[28]

11C-acetate accumulates in primary invasive transitional cell carcinoma (TCC) of the urinary bladder and metastatic nodes. False-positive accumulation may occur at sites of inflammation, in particular in patients pretreated with Bacillus-Calmette-Guérin (BCG). In contrast, in non-BCG–exposed patients with invasive TCC, including patients treated with neoadjuvant chemotherapy, 11C-acetate PET/CT may play a useful role in staging.[28]

REFERENCES

1. Grassi I, Nanni C, Allegri V, et al. The clinical use of PET with 11C-acetate. Am J Nucl Med Mol Imaging 2012;2(1):33–47.

2. Ohtsuka T, Nomori H, Watanabe K, et al. Positive imaging of thymoma by 11C-acetate positron emission tomography. Ann Thorac Surg 2006;81:1132–4.

3. Lee SM, Kim TS, Kim SK. Cerebellopontine angle schwannoma on 11C-acetate PET/CT. Clin Nucl Med 2009;34:831–3.

4. Ho CL, Chen S, Ho KM, et al. 11C-acetate PET/CT in multicentric angiomyolipoma of the kidney. Clin Nucl Med 2011;36:407–8.

5. Wang HC, Zhao J, Zuo CT, et al. Encephalitis depicted by a combination of 11C-acetate and F-18 FDG PET/CT. Clin Nucl Med 2009;34:952–4.

6. Lee SM, Kim TS, Lee JW, et al. Incidental finding of an 11C-acetate PET-positive multiple myeloma. Ann Nucl Med 2010;24:41–4.

7. Swinnen JV, Heemers H, Deboel L, et al. Stimulation of tumor-associated fatty acid synthase expression by growth factor activation of the sterol regulatory element-binding protein pathway. Oncogene 2000; 19:5173–81.

8. Swinnen JV, Van Veldhoven PP, Timmermans L, et al. Fatty acid synthase drives the synthesis of phospholipids partitioning into detergent-resistant membrane microdomains. Biochem Biophys Res Commun 2003;302:898–903.

9. Seltzer MA, Jahan SA, Sparks R, et al. Radiation dose estimates in humans for (11)C-acetate whole-body PET. J Nucl Med 2004;45:1233–6.

10. Cerdan S, Kunnecke B, Seelig J. Cerebral metabolism of [1,2-13C]acetate as detected by in vivo and in vitro 13C NMR. J Biol Chem 1990;265: 12916–26.

11. Yoshimoto M, Waki A, Yonekura Y, et al. Characterization of acetate metabolism in tumor cells in relation to cell proliferation: acetate metabolism in tumor cells. Nucl Med Biol 2001;28:117–22.

12. Liu RS, Chang CP, Guo WY, et al. 11C-acetate versus 18F-FDG PET in detection of meningioma and monitoring the effect of gamma-knife radiosurgery. J Nucl Med 2010;51:883–91.

13. Buchegger F, Garibotto V, Zilli T, et al. First imaging results of an intraindividual comparison of 11C-acetate and 18F-fluorocholine PET/CT in patients with prostate cancer at early biochemical first or second relapse after prostatectomy or radiotherapy. Eur J Nucl Med Mol Imaging 2014;41:68–78.

14. Wachter S, Tomek S, Kurtaran A, et al. 11C-Acetate positron emission tomography imaging and image fusion with computed tomography and magnetic resonance imaging in patients with recurrent prostate cancer. J Clin Oncol 2006;24:2513–9.

15. Yeh SH, Liu RS, Wu LC, et al. 11C-acetate clearance in nasopharyngeal carcinoma. Nucl Med Commun 1999;20:131–4.

16. Sun A, Sörensen J, Karlsson M, et al. 1-[11C]-acetate PET imaging in head and neck cancer—a comparison with 18F-FDG-PET: implications for staging and radiotherapy planning. Eur J Nucl Med Mol Imaging 2007;34:651–7.

17. Nomori H, Shibata H, Uno K, et al. 11C-acetate can be used in place of 18F-fluorodeoxyglucose for positron emission tomography imaging of non-small cell lung cancer with higher sensitivity for well differentiated adenocarcinoma. J Thorac Oncol 2008;3:1427–32.

18. Shreve PD, Gross MD. Imaging of the pancreas and related diseases with PET carbon-11-acetate. J Nucl Med 1997;38:1305–10.

19. Huo L, Wu Z, Zhuang H, et al. Dual time point 11C-acetate PET imaging can potentially distinguish focal nodular hyperplasia from primary hepatocellular carcinoma. Clin Nucl Med 2009;34:874–7.

20. Ho CL, Yu SC, Yeung DW. 11C-acetate PET imaging in hepatocellular carcinoma and other liver masses. J Nucl Med 2003;44:213–21.

21. Sandblom G, Sörensen J, Lundin N, et al. Positron emission tomography with C11-acetate for tumor detection and localization in patients with prostate-specific antigen relapse after radical prostatectomy. Urology 2006;67(5):996–1000.

22. Shreve P, Chiao PC, Humes HD, et al. 11C-acetate PET imaging in renal disease. J Nucl Med 1995; 36:1595–601.

23. Brogsitter C, Zöphel K, Kotzerke J. 18F-Choline, 11C-choline and 11C-acetate PET/CT: comparative analysis for imaging prostate cancer patients. Eur J Nucl Med Mol Imaging 2013;40(Suppl 1):S18–27.

24. Schiepers C, Hoh CK, Nuyts J, et al. 1-11C-acetate kinetics of prostate cancer. J Nucl Med 2008;49: 206–15.

25. Mena E, Turkbey B, Mani H, et al. 11C-Acetate PET/CT in localized prostate cancer: a study with MRI and histopathologic correlation. J Nucl Med 2012; 53:538–45.

26. Jambor I, Borra R, Kemppainen J, et al. Functional imaging of localized prostate cancer aggressiveness using 11C-acetate PET/CT and 1H-MR spectroscopy. J Nucl Med 2010;51:1676–83.

27. Hara T, Bansal A, DeGrado TR. Effect of hypoxia on the uptake of [methyl-3H]choline, [1-14C] acetate and [18F]FDG in cultured prostate cancer cells. Nucl Med Biol 2006;33:977–84.

28. Schöder H, Ong SC, Reuter VE, et al. Initial results with 11C-acetate positron emission tomography/computed tomography (PET/CT) in the staging of urinary bladder cancer. Mol Imaging Biol 2012;14:245–51.

PET/MRI Radiotracer Beyond ^{18}F-FDG

Miguel Hernandez Pampaloni, MD, PhD[a],*, Lorenzo Nardo, MD[a,b]

KEYWORDS

• PET • MRI • Imaging • Radiotracers

KEY POINTS

• The recent development and introduction of new hybrid imaging devices combining positron emission tomography (PET) technology with magnetic resonance imaging (MRI) opens up new perspectives in clinical molecular imaging.
• Combining MRI and fluorine-18 choline PET would theoretically produce valuable clinical data in a single imaging session, which can be used for staging, prognosis, and assessment of treatment response.
• Fluorine-18–sodium fluoride (18F-NaF) is a highly sensitive PET tracer used as a marker of osteoblastic abnormalities.
• PET imaging with ^{68}Ga–tetraazacyclododecane tetraacetic acid–octreotate (^{68}Ga-DOTATATE) or [^{68}Ga]-DOTA-D Phe^1-Tyr^3-Octreotide (DOTATOC) has demonstrated promising results for locating metastatic lesions, occasionally with superior sensitivity than whole-body MRI.
• 3,4-diidrossi-L-fenilalanina (L-DOPA) PET adds data regarding L-DOPA metabolism, which may increase the specificity and sensibility of the study itself.
• Fluoromisonidazole is known to be not only a useful tracer for determining hypoxic cells but also an efficient hypoxic radiosensitizer.

INTRODUCTION

Positron emission tomography (PET) has contributed significantly in the past 2 decades to the advances of understanding the physiology and pathophysiology of a variety of biologic processes in cardiology, neurosciences, and oncology. In combination with computed tomography (CT), PET/CT imaging has evolved into the cornerstone of oncologic imaging in the past decade, becoming standard of care in the staging, characterization, and assessment of treatment response for many solid tumors. The recent development and market introduction of new hybrid imaging devices, combining PET technology with magnetic resonance imaging (MRI), opens new perspectives in clinical molecular imaging. The intrinsic superior soft tissue contrast of MRI compared with CT and the lack of ionizing radiation are obvious advantages of this new technology. Although fluorine-18 fluorodeoxyglucose (18F-FDG) remains the pivotal radiopharmaceutical used clinically, an increasing number of other PET imaging probes have also been used in the clinical and research settings. This article describes some of the current radiopharmaceuticals beyond FDG that can be used with PET/MRI imaging, rather than enumerating all the ongoing research regarding molecular imaging PET probes.

FLUORINE-18 CHOLINE/CARBON-11 CHOLINE

Choline is an amino acid needed for the synthesis of phospholipids in cell membranes, methyl metabolism, cholinergic neurotransmission, transmembrane signaling, and lipid-cholesterol transport and

^{a} Department of Radiology and Biomedical Imaging, University of California, 505 Parnassus Avenue, M-396, San Francisco, CA 94143, USA; ^{b} Department of Radiology, Brescia, Italy
* Corresponding author.
E-mail address: miguel.pampaloni@ucsf.edu

PET Clin 9 (2014) 345–349
http://dx.doi.org/10.1016/j.cpet.2014.03.010

metabolism. The most important metabolic process for the tumor detection is the aberrant phospholipid metabolism (upregulation of choline kinase), which results in an increased mitotic signaling and plasma membrane biosynthesis.[1] Choline is transported inside the cell, phosphorylated, and metabolized to phosphatidylcholine, as described by the Kennedy pathway.[2] The use of radiolabeled choline compounds has been shown to be of use for detecting recurrences of numerous solid tumors, such as prostate, brain, lung, and bladder cancers. Different choline compounds have been studied and several efforts have been made to improve the imaging quality of the radiopharmaceutical, especially regarding its degradation to betaine and its physical half-life.[3] Some compounds, such as 18F-fluoromethyl-[1,2-2H4]-choline (18F-D4-FCH), are more resistant to its oxidation than betaine. Regarding the half-life, 11C-choline requires the presence of a cyclotron because of the short half-life (20.4 minutes), whereas fluorinated compounds have a longer half-life (109.8 minutes) and can transfer more easily.

The larger body of literature to date describes the application of choline radiopharmaceuticals in prostate cancer and brain tumors. In the prostate, the main advantage offered by MRI is a more accurate visualization of small pelvic anatomic structures and reliable localization of intraprostate and bone lesions when compared with CT.[4] 18F-choline localizes not only in the malignant tissue but also in normal tissues, such as bowel and ureters. The simultaneous use of PET/MRI might increase the accuracy of prostate tumor detection within the prostate gland and in regional and distant locations, such as lymph node or bones. Furthermore, PET/MRI with 18F-choline might also have a role in detecting early biochemical recurrence and in external-beam radiotherapy planning.

In brain tumors, 18F-choline accumulates in the neoplastic tissue and accurately differentiates it from normal brain parenchyma.[5] Magnetic resonance imaging is standard of care and allows spectroscopy analysis and diffusion sequences to be performed, which provide functional and metabolic information. Combining MRI and 18F-choline PET would theoretically produce valuable clinical data in a single imaging session, which can be used for staging, prognosis, and assessment of treatment response.

GALLIUM 68–TETRAAZACYCLODODECANE TETRAACETIC ACID–OCTREOTATE COMPOUNDS

Gallium 68–tetraazacyclododecane tetraacetic acid–octreotate (^{68}Ga-DOTATATE) is an amide of

the acid 1,4,7,10-tetraazacyclododecane-1,4,7,10-tetraacetic acid (DOTA), which binds a derivative of octreotide (Tyr)-octreotate.[6] Similar molecules are [^{68}Ga]-DOTA-D Phe[1]-Tyr[3]-Octreotide (^{68}Ga-DOTATOC) (DOTA-D-phel-Tyr3-octreotide) and DOTANOC (DOTA-1-Nal-octreotide). The use of these radiotracers has recently increased because of their convenient preparation using a germanium-68/gallium-68 (68Ge/68Ga) generator. The final octreotide compound binds selectively to somatostatin receptor type 2 (SSTR), which is characteristically highly expressed by neuroendocrine tumor cells.[7] Somatostatin receptor type 2 has several major subtypes and, because of the unequal distribution of them in SSTR-positive malignancies, the structures of the somatostatin analogs varied to obtain high binding affinity.

It has been already demonstrated that PET imaging with somatostatin analogs is superior over more conventional imaging and single photon imaging tomography with 111-Indium (^{111}In)-pentetreotide, with a positive effect on patient treatment and prognostic accuracy.[8] Because of the phenotypic behavior of recurrent neuroendocrine tumor (NET), PET imaging with ^{68}Ga–tetraazacyclododecane tetraacetic acid–octreotate (^{68}Ga-DOTATATE) or DOTATOC has shown promising results for locating metastatic lesions, occasionally with superior sensitivity than whole-body MRI.[9] The high sensitivity of this radiotracer combined with the image resolution of the MRI will present a powerful diagnostic tool, especially for diagnosing tumor recurrence and detecting metastasis. Recent studies have reported the presence of SSTRs within benign tumors,[10] and the integration of the radiotracer with the robust MRI image resolution may increase testing specificity.

FLUORINE-18–SODIUM FLUORIDE

Fluorine-18–sodium fluoride (18F-NaF) is a highly sensitive PET tracer used for detecting skeletal osteoblastic abnormalities.[11,12] Fluorine-18–sodium fluoride is an analog of the hydroxyl ion in the bone matrix and is rapidly exchanged with high initial extraction fraction in the hydroxyapatite crystals. The uptake of 18F-NaF correlates with blood flow and bone remodeling; therefore, it is not tumor-specific and can be a viable option for studying different benign skeletal processes.[13] Initial 18F-NaF applications have targeted processes in pediatric and adult populations based on the paradigm of measuring osteoblastic activity and bone turnover.[14] Some recent studies have shown increased sensitivity with 18F-NaF PET/CT compared with MRI, especially for detecting osteoblastic bone metastasis.[15] Preliminary data on the combined use of PET/MRI seem to suggest that the 18F-NaF–increased PET sensitivity and robust MRI specificity will present a valuable tool for the early diagnosis of osteoblastic bone metastasis and the assessment of treatment response.[16]

FLUORINE-18–LABELED DIHYDROXYPHENYLALANINE

Dihydroxyphenylalanine (DOPA) is a neutral amino acid analog to the dopamine precursor 3,4-dihydroxy-L-phenylalanine (L-DOPA). It is internalized by the amino acid transport system for large neutral amino acids and enters the catecholamine metabolic pathway of endogenous L-DOPA in the brain and peripheral tissue.[17] It was first assembled with 18F for the study of Parkinson disease. Its use has recently been expanded to include imaging of some neuroendocrine tumors, primary brain neoplasias, and pancreatic cell hyperplasia.[18,19] All of these disorders share an increased activity of L-DOPA decarboxylase, and therefore demonstrate high uptake of 18F-DOPA. Once injected, 18F-DOPA is physiologically distributed in the basal ganglia, pancreas, and adrenal glands and excreted by the liver and kidneys.[17] Recent studies showed a clinical use of L-DOPA PET scan in distinguishing high-grade and low-grade brain tumors and tumor tissue, with high-grade tumors being more L-DOPA–avid than lower-grade tumors[20]; and in the same fashion, L-DOPA PET can differentiate tumor tissue from post–radiation therapy changes.[21] It is easy to imagine how the fusion of this technique with MRI can boost the diagnosis and follow-up of brain tumors. MRI can provide high-resolution morphologic detail along with important specific quantitative imaging biomarkers, such as index of diffusion (diffusion-weighted imaging), perfusion (Dynamic Contrast Enhancement [DCE]-MRI), and metabolic analysis (spectroscopy), within the tissue and hypoxia (texture analysis and Blood-oxygen-level-dependent [BOLD]); on the other hand, L-DOPA PET adds data regarding L-DOPA metabolism, which may increase the specificity and sensibility of the study itself.

FLUORINE-18–FLUTEMETAMOL

Flutemetamol (2-[4-(methylamino)phenyl]-1,3-benzothiazol-6-ol) is a neutral analog of thioflavin T. Multiple studies have confirmed the capability of this molecule to cross the blood–brain barrier and to reversibly bind fibrillar β-amyloid in the brain.[22]

Flutemetamol was initially labeled with an 11C isotope, limiting its availability because of the 20-minute half-life of the 11C. 18-Florbetapir is a similar agent, which tracks the amyloid deposits and has shown some promise in assessing the β-amyloid protein involved in the development of Alzheimer-type dementia.[23] The increased accessibility to these components, along with their important clinical significance, should benefit the use of PET/MRI in this area. Combined PET/MRI may become a valuable research and clinical tool to noninvasively evaluate neurologic processes using the integrated morphologic and biochemical information offered by this technology.

FLUORINE-18–FLUOROMISONIDAZOLE

Fluorine-18–fluoromisonidazole (F-MISO) is one of the most commonly used radiotracer for hypoxia. Misonidazole is a nitroimidazole and thus, after passive diffusion into the cell, is reduced with nitro anion radicals. In the presence of oxygen, the last reaction is reversible and the molecule can leave the cell, but in absence of oxygen, misonidazole is reduced and remains trapped in the cell.

Since the early 1980s, Misonidazole has been known to be not only a useful tracer for identifying hypoxic cells but also an efficient hypoxic radiosensitizer.[24] Because of the relationship between hypoxia and treatment resistance, this radiotracer can be used to monitor tumor volume and hypoxia in different tumors, such as glioblastoma, head and neck tumors, and all tumors that are treated with radiotherapy.[25] F-MISO have been studied also with respect to other neurologic applications, for example stroke.

Furthermore, F-MISO can be a sensitive tool for the noninvasive quantification of hypoxia in cardiac tissue and can have valuable cardiologic applications.[26] For example, it might be clinically used in the study of myocardial ischemia, myocardial hibernation, cardiomyopathies, vascular collateral development, and response to revascularization procedures. All of these neurologic and cardiologic applications of F-MISO might be improved by combining it with MRI, especially multimodal MRI, including carbogen breathing during BOLD MRI, which can accurately and noninvasively detect hypoxia. The hypoxia study would greatly benefit from the fusion of MRI and PET.

CARDIOVASCULAR MOLECULAR IMAGING APPLICATIONS

Positron emission tomography allows an accurate assessment of myocardial perfusion and coronary artery disease (CAD), and remains a valuable tool for the assessing myocardial viability in patients with severe left ventricular dysfunction. Positron emission tomography/computed tomography imaging allows a comprehensive evaluation of the functional and morphologic severity of CAD. Combining the ability of MRI to produce high-resolution anatomic images and the high sensitivity of PET for detecting molecular targets may help extend these modalities into new applications, including atherosclerotic plaque characterization, stem cell tracking, and evaluation of angiogenesis.

Fluorine-18–FDG is an excellent marker for glucose disposal rate and has already been used to image early inflammatory changes in the endothelial vascular lumen as surrogate markers of preclinical atherosclerotic disease. Inflammation has been known to be a component of the reparative process after an ischemic insult, and formation of new capillaries occurs in response to ischemia. Tumor angiogenesis has been described as a possible biomarker for diagnosis, treatment, and evaluation of response to therapy. Specific proteins that behave as receptors, such as AvB5 integrin and AvB3 integrin are overexpressed in new active endothelial cells and represent a marker of neoangiogenesis. 18F-fluciclatide[27] is a marker of neoangiogenesis given its high affinity for binding AvB3 integrin and AvB5 integrin, and some solid tumors have already been shown to express AvB3 and AvB5 integrins more than others. In combination with high anatomic MRI resolution, the localization of these new vessel formations would be able to be assessed more accurately.

The sympathetic nervous system has been studied with several PET radiopharmaceuticals, such as the catecholamine analog 11C-labeled meta-hydroxyephedrine, which may be used to assess abnormalities in myocardial sympathetic innervation caused by various cardiac diseases, such as CAD, heart failure, and arrhythmogenic disorders.[28] It seems logical that the combination of PET and MRI might facilitate risk stratification, and it may help to focus on areas of studies in which innervation plays an important role, such as electric disorders or myocardial infarctions.[29]

REFERENCES

1. Katz-Brull R, Seger D, Rivenson-Segal D, et al. Metabolic markers of breast cancer: enhanced choline metabolism and reduced choline-ether-phospholipid synthesis. Cancer Res 2002;62(7): 1966–70.
2. Fernandez-Murray JP, McMaster CR. Glycerophosphocholine catabolism as a new route for choline formation for phosphatidylcholine synthesis by the Kennedy pathway. J Biol Chem 2005;280(46): 38290–6. http://dx.doi.org/10.1074/jbc.M507700200.
3. Witney TH, Alam IS, Turton DR, et al. Evaluation of deuterated 18F- and 11C-labeled choline analogs for cancer detection by positron emission tomography. Clin Cancer Res 2012;18(4):1063–72. http://dx.doi.org/10.1158/1078-0432.CCR-11-2462.
4. Wetter A, Lipponer C, Nensa F, et al. Evaluation of the PET component of simultaneous [(18)F]choline PET/MRI in prostate cancer: comparison with [(18)F]choline PET/CT. Eur J Nucl Med Mol Imaging 2014; 41(1):79–88. http://dx.doi.org/10.1007/s00259-013-2560-2.
5. Shinoura N, Nishijima M, Hara T, et al. Brain tumors: detection with C-11 choline PET. Radiology 1997; 202(2):497–503. http://dx.doi.org/10.1148/radiology.202.2.9015080.
6. Eisenwiener KP, Prata MI, Buschmann I, et al. NODAGATOC, a new chelator-coupled somatostatin analogue labeled with [67/68Ga] and [111In] for SPECT, PET, and targeted therapeutic applications of somatostatin receptor (hsst2) expressing tumors. Bioconjug Chem 2002;13(3):530–41.
7. Mayerhoefer ME, Ba-Ssalamah A, Weber M, et al. Gadoxetate-enhanced versus diffusion-weighted MRI for fused Ga-68-DOTANOC PET/MRI in patients with neuroendocrine tumours of the upper abdomen. Eur Radiol 2013;23(7):1978–85. http://dx.doi.org/10.1007/s00330-013-2785-2.
8. Bhate K, Mok WY, Tran K, et al. Functional assessment in the multimodality imaging of pancreatic neuro-endocrine tumours. Minerva Endocrinol 2010; 35(1):17–25.
9. Putzer D, Gabriel M, Henninger B, et al. Bone metastases in patients with neuroendocrine tumor: 68Ga-DOTA-Tyr3-octreotide PET in comparison to CT and bone scintigraphy. J Nucl Med 2009;50(8):1214–21. http://dx.doi.org/10.2967/jnumed.108.060236.
10. Kuyumcu S, Ozkan ZG, Sanli Y, et al. Physiological and tumoral uptake of (68)Ga-DOTATATE: standardized uptake values and challenges in interpretation. Ann Nucl Med 2013;27(6):538–45. http://dx.doi.org/10.1007/s12149-013-0718-4.
11. Czernin J, Satyamurthy N, Schiepers C. Molecular mechanisms of bone 18F-NaF deposition. J Nucl Med 2010;51(12):1826–9. http://dx.doi.org/10.2967/jnumed.110.077933.
12. Poulsen MH, Petersen H, Hoilund-Carlsen PF, et al. Spine metastases in prostate cancer: comparison of [99mTc]MDP wholebody bone scintigraphy, [18F]choline PET/CT, and [18F]NaF PET/CT. BJU Int 2013. http://dx.doi.org/10.1111/bju.12599.
13. Desai B, Gross ME, Jadvar H. Multimodality imaging in biochemical recurrence of prostate cancer: utility of (18)F-NaF PET/CT in early detection of metastasis. Rev Esp Med Nucl Imagen Mol 2012;31(4):231–2. http://dx.doi.org/10.1016/j.remn.2012.03.008.

14. Li Y, Schiepers C, Lake R, et al. Clinical utility of (18) F-fluoride PET/CT in benign and malignant bone diseases. Bone 2012;50(1):128–39. http://dx.doi.org/10.1016/j.bone.2011.09.053.

15. Mosavi F, Johansson S, Sandberg DT, et al. Whole-body diffusion-weighted MRI compared with (18)F-NaF PET/CT for detection of bone metastases in patients with high-risk prostate carcinoma. AJR Am J Roentgenol 2012;199(5):1114–20. http://dx.doi.org/10.2214/AJR.11.8351.

16. Ouvrier MJ, Vignot S, Thariat J. State of the art in nuclear imaging for the diagnosis of bone metastases. Bull Cancer 2013;100(11):1115–24. http://dx.doi.org/10.1684/bdc.2013.1847 [in French].

17. Chondrogiannis S, Marzola MC, Al-Nahhas A, et al. Normal biodistribution pattern and physiologic variants of 18F-DOPA PET imaging. Nucl Med Commun 2013;34(12):1141–9. http://dx.doi.org/10.1097/MNM.0000000000000008.

18. Youland RS, Kitange GJ, Peterson TE, et al. The role of LAT1 in (18)F-DOPA uptake in malignant gliomas. J Neurooncol 2013;111(1):11–8. http://dx.doi.org/10.1007/s11060-012-0986-1.

19. Yang J, Yuan L, Meeks JK, et al. 18F-DOPA positron emission tomography/computed tomography application in congenital hyperinsulinism. J Pediatr Endocrinol Metab 2012;25(7–8):619–22. http://dx.doi.org/10.1515/jpem-2012-0114.

20. Nioche C, Soret M, Gontier E, et al. Evaluation of quantitative criteria for glioma grading with static and dynamic 18F-FDopa PET/CT. Clin Nucl Med 2013;38(2):81–7. http://dx.doi.org/10.1097/RLU.0b013e318279fd5a.

21. Lizarraga KJ, Allen-Auerbach M, Czernin J, et al. 18F-FDOPA PET for differentiating recurrent or progressive brain metastatic tumors from late or delayed radiation injury after radiation treatment. J Nucl Med 2014;55(1):30–6. http://dx.doi.org/10.2967/jnumed.113.121418.

22. Mason NS, Mathis CA, Klunk WE. Positron emission tomography radioligands for in vivo imaging of Aβ plaques. J Labelled Comp Radiopharm 2013;56(3–4):89–95. http://dx.doi.org/10.1002/jlcr.2989.

23. Leinonen V, Rinne JO, Virtanen KA, et al. Positron emission tomography with [18F]flutemetamol and [11C]PiB for in vivo detection of cerebral cortical amyloid in normal pressure hydrocephalus patients. Eur J Neurol 2013;20(7):1043–52. http://dx.doi.org/10.1111/ene.12102.

24. Asquith JC, Watts ME, Patel K, et al. Electron affinic sensitization. V. Radiosensitization of hypoxic bacteria and mammalian cells in vitro by some nitroimidazoles and nitropyrazoles. Radiat Res 1974;60(1):108–18.

25. Tachibana I, Nishimura Y, Shibata T, et al. A prospective clinical trial of tumor hypoxia imaging with 18F-fluoromisonidazole positron emission tomography and computed tomography (F-MISO PET/CT) before and during radiation therapy. J Radiat Res 2013;54(6):1078–84. http://dx.doi.org/10.1093/jrr/rrt033.

26. Handley MG, Medina RA, Nagel E, et al. PET imaging of cardiac hypoxia: opportunities and challenges. J Mol Cell Cardiol 2011;51(5):640–50. http://dx.doi.org/10.1016/j.yjmcc.2011.07.005.

27. Battle MR, Goggi JL, Allen L, et al. Monitoring tumor response to antiangiogenic sunitinib therapy with 18F-fluciclatide, an 18F-labeled alphaVbeta3-integrin and alphaV beta5-integrin imaging agent. J Nucl Med 2011;52(3):424–30. http://dx.doi.org/10.2967/jnumed.110.077479.

28. Caldwell JH, Link JM, Levy WC, et al. Evidence for pre- to postsynaptic mismatch of the cardiac sympathetic nervous system in ischemic congestive heart failure. J Nucl Med 2008;49:234–41.

29. Saraste A, Nekolla SG, Schwaiger M. Cardiovascular molecular imaging: an overview. Cardiovasc Res 2009;83(4):643–52.

Index

Note: Page numbers of article titles are in **boldface** type.

A

Abdomen
    ^{11}C-acetate imaging for, 341–342
    ^{18}F-fluorocholine imaging for, 301–303
    ^{18}F-fluoro-DOPA imaging for, 313–314
    ^{18}F-fluorothymidine imaging for, 334–335
    gallium-68 labeled somatostatin receptor imaging
        for, 327
Abscess, brain, 273
Acetabulum, defects of, 282
^{11}C-Acetate, **339–344**
    for abdomen imaging, 341–342
    for central nervous system imaging, 340
    for head and neck imaging, 340
    for pelvis imaging, 342–343
    for thorax imaging, 340–341
Acetylcholine synthesis, 300
Adrenal glands
    ^{18}F-fluorocholine imaging for, 302–303
    ^{18}F-fluoro-DOPA imaging for, 313
Aging
    ^{18}F-fluorothymidine uptake and, 335
    gallium-68 labeled somatostatin receptor uptake
        and, 327
Alzheimer dementia, 267–270, 347
Amyloid imaging, 268, 270, 347
Angiogenesis, ^{18}F-fluoromisonidazole imaging
    for, 348
Ankylosing spondylitis, 280
AvB5 integrin, 348

B

Back pain, 279–280, 288–292
Bisphosphonate therapy, 283
Bladder, ^{11}C-acetate imaging for, 343
Bone
    cancer of, 294
    ^{18}F-fluoride imaging for, **277–285, 287–297,**
        346–347
    ^{18}F-fluorothymidine imaging for, 333
    osteoblastic abnormalities of, 346–347
    viability of, 293–294
Bone grafts, 282
Brain
    ^{18}F-fluoro-DOPA imaging for, 312–313, 347
    nonmalignant conditions of, **267–276**
Brain tumors
    ^{11}C-acetate imaging for, 340
    ^{18}F-dihydroxyphenylalanine imaging for, 347
    ^{18}F-fluorocholine imaging for, 300
    ^{18}F-fluoro-DOPA imaging for, 308
    ^{18}F-fluorothymidine imaging for, 332–333
    ^{11}C-methionine imaging for, 261–264
    radiotracers for, 272–273
Bronchioalveolar cell carcinoma, 301

C

Cancer
    bone, 294
    ^{18}F-fluorothymidine imaging for, **331–338**
    gastric, 335
    lung, 301
    prostate. See Prostate, cancer of.
Carbidopa, for premedication, in ^{18}F-fluoro-DOPA
    imaging, 309–314
Carcinoid tumors, ^{18}F-fluoro-DOPA imaging for,
    308–309, 312, 317
Cardiovascular disorders
    ^{18}F-fluoromisonidazole imaging for, 347–348
    PET/MRI imaging for, 347–348
Central nervous system. See also Brain; |Brain
    tumors.
    ^{11}C-acetate imaging for, 340
    ^{18}F-fluorocholine imaging for, 300–301
Cervical cages, 280
Chemotherapy, ^{18}F-fluorothymidine uptake and,
    335–336
Child abuse, fractures in, 283, 294
Cholangiocarcinoma, 341
^{11}C-Choline, 299
    for PET/MRI, 345–346
    procedures for, 264–265
^{18}F-Choline. See ^{18}F-Fluorocholine.
Clinical Trials Network, standardization programs
    of, 260
Cognitive impairment, 268, 270
Colchicine, ^{18}F-fluorocholine imaging interactions
    with, 304
Colon, ^{18}F-fluorocholine imaging for, 302
Condylar hyperplasia, 279
Coronary artery disease, 347–348

D

Dementia, 267–270, 347
    with Lewy bodies, 268

PET Clin 9 (2014) 351–354
http://dx.doi.org/10.1016/S1556-8598(14)00047-9
1556-8598/14/$ – see front matter © 2014 Elsevier Inc. All rights reserved.

Demyelination, 273
Dentures, maladaptive, 279
^{18}F-Dihydroxyphenylalanine. *see* ^{18}F-Fluoro-DOPA.
Dynamic Contrast Enhancement, 347

E

Epilepsy, 270
^{18}F-Ethyl choline, 299
European Association of Nuclear Medicine,
    standardization programs of, 259–260
European Organisation for Research and Treatment
    of Cancer Imaging Group, standardization
    programs of, 260
Ewing sarcoma, 294

F

^{18}F-Florbetaben, for brain disorders, 267
^{18}F-Florbetapir, for brain disorders, 267–268, 347
^{11}C-Flumazenil, for brain disorders, 268–270, 273
^{18}F-Flumazenil, for brain disorders, 268–270
^{18}F-Flumetamol
    for brain disorders, 267, 347
    for PET/MRI, 347
^{18}F-Fluoride. *See* ^{18}F-Sodium fluoride.
^{18}F-Fluorocholine
    drug effects on, 304–305
    for abdomen imaging, 301–303
    for central nervous system disorders, 300–301
    for genitourinary system imaging, 303
    for head and neck imaging, 300–301
    for pelvis imaging, 303
    for PET/MRI, 345–346
    for thorax imaging, 301
    tracers based on, 299
^{18}F-Fluoro-DOPA, **307–321**
    acquisition protocol for, 309–310
    clinical applications of, 308–309
    for brain disorders, 268–269, 271, 273
    for PET/MRI, 347
    normal distribution of, 310–311
    pitfalls involving, 314–319
    premedication effects on, 309–314
    structure of, 308
^{18}F-Fluoroethyltyrosine, for brain disorders, 269,
    272–273
^{18}F-Fluoromethylcholine, for PET/MRI, 346
^{18}F-Fluoromisonidazole, for PET/MRI, 347
^{18}F-Fluoropropyl dihydrotetrabenazine, for brain
    disorders, 268–269, 271
^{18}F-Fluorothymidine
    for brain disorders, 268–269, 273
    for proliferation imaging, **331–339**
        aging effects on, 335
        in abdomen, 334–335
        in genitourinary system, 335

        in head and neck, 332–333
        in pelvis, 335
        in thorax, 334
        treatment effects on, 335–336
Focal nodular hyperplasia, of liver, 341
Foot pain, 282
Fractures, in children, 292–294
Frontotemporal dementia, 268

G

Gallbladder, ^{18}F-fluoro-DOPA imaging for, 315
Gallium-68 labeled somatostatin receptors, **323–329**
    chemical structures of, 323
    clinical background of, 323–325
    factors affecting imaging results, 327
    for PET/MRI, 346
    imaging guidelines for, 325–327
Gallium-68 Users Group, standardized programs
    of, 260
Gastrointestinal system
    ^{18}F-fluorocholine imaging for, 302
    ^{18}F-fluorothymidine imaging for, 335
^{18}F-GE-180, for brain disorders, 274
Genitourinary system
    ^{18}F-fluorocholine imaging for, 303
    ^{18}F-fluoro-DOPA imaging for, 315
    ^{18}F-fluorothymidine imaging for, 335
Germanium-68, for gallium-68 labeled somatostatin
    receptor preparation, 324
Glioblastomas
    ^{11}C-acetate imaging for, 340
    ^{18}F-fluorocholine imaging for, 300
Gliomas, 273
    ^{18}F-fluorothymidine imaging for, 332
    ^{11}C-methionine imaging for, 261

H

"Harmonized PET Reconstructions for Cancer
    Clinical Trials," 260
Head and neck
    ^{11}C-acetate imaging for, 340
    cancer of, 332–333
    ^{18}F-fluorocholine imaging for, 300–301
    ^{18}F-fluoro-DOPA imaging for, 312–315
    ^{18}F-fluorothymidine imaging for, 333
    gallium-68 labeled somatostatin receptor imaging
        for, 327
Hemangiomas, of liver, 341
Hepatocellular carcinoma, 302
Hepatomas, 302
Hip, ^{18}F-sodium fluoride uptake in, 281–282
Hormone replacement therapy, ^{18}F-fluorocholine
    imaging interactions with, 304–305
^{11}C-Hydroxyepinephrine, for cardiovascular
    imaging, 348

Hyperinsulinemic hypoglycemia, ^{18}F-fluoro-DOPA imaging forH, 309, 316
Hyperostosis cranialis interna, 279
Hypoxia, 347

I

Inflammation, brain, radiotracers for, 273–274
Insulinomas, 309, 312
Intestine, ^{11}C-acetate imaging for, 343
Ischemia, ^{18}F-fluoromisonidazole imaging for, 347
Ischiopubic synchondrosis, bone turnover at, 292

J

Japanese Society of Nuclear Medicine, standardization programs of, 260–261
Jaw, ^{18}F-sodium fluoride uptake in, 279

K

Kidney
    ^{11}C-acetate imaging for, 341–342
    ^{18}F-fluorocholine imaging for, 303
    ^{18}F-fluoro-DOPA imaging for, 315
    ^{18}F-fluorothymidine imaging for, 335
    ^{18}F-sodium fluoride uptake in, 279
Knee, ligament injury in, 282–283

L

Langerhans cell histiocytosis, 293
Leg, ^{18}F-sodium fluoride uptake in, 282
Leukoencephalitis, 273
Liver
    ^{11}C-acetate imaging for, 341–342
    ^{18}F-fluorocholine imaging for, 302
    ^{18}F-fluorothymidine imaging for, 334–335
L-type amino acid transporter, 272
Lung
    ^{11}C-acetate imaging for, 340–341
    cancer of, 301
    ^{18}F-fluorocholine imaging for, 301
Lutetium-177, for gallium-68 labeled somatostatin receptor preparation, 324
Lymph nodes
    ^{18}F-fluorocholine imaging for, 303
    ^{18}F-fluorothymidine imaging for, 332–333
Lymphadenopathy, of mediastinum, 340–341
Lymphoma, 333

M

Magnetic resonance imaging, for brain tumors, 273
Maxillary sinus, ^{18}F-fluorocholine imaging for, 300
Meningiomas
    ^{11}C-acetate imaging for, 340
    ^{18}F-fluorocholine imaging for, 300
Mesothelioma, 301
Metastasis, to bone, 279, 294

^{11}C-Methionine
    for brain disorders, 272–273
    procedures for, 261–264
^{11}C-Methyl tryptophan, for brain disorders, 270
^{18}F-Methylcholine, 299–300
Microcytomas, 308–309
Microglia, activation of, in inflammation, 273–274
Movement disorders, 270–272
Multiple endocrine neoplasia, 309
Multiple myeloma, 279
Multiple sclerosis, 274
Myocardial ischemia, 347

N

Neuroblastomas, 294, 309
Neuroendocrine tumors
    ^{18}F-fluoro-DOPA imaging for, 308–309, 347
    gallium-68 compound imaging for, 323–327, 346
Neuroinflammation, radiotracers for, 273–274

O

Oligodendrogliomas, 273
Osteoarthritis, of foot, 282
Osteoblastomas, 293
Osteoid osteomas, 280, 293
Osteonecrosis, 279
Osteoporosis, 283, 293
Osteosarcomas, 294
Otomastoiditis, 301

P

Paget disease, 279, 283, 293
Pancreas
    ^{11}C-acetate imaging for, 341–342
    B-cell hyperplasia of, 309
    cell hyperplasia in, 347
    ^{18}F-fluorocholine imaging for, 302
    ^{18}F-fluoro-DOPA imaging for, 311–312, 315–318, 347
    gallium-68 labeled somatostatin receptor imaging for, 326
Paragangliomas, 308–310, 314, 316–318
Parathyroid gland, ^{18}F-fluorocholine imaging for, 300
Parkinson disease, 271–272, 308, 347
Parotid gland, ^{18}F-fluorocholine imaging for, 300
^{11}C-PBR-28, for brain disorders, 274
Pediatric patients, ^{18}F-sodium fluoride imaging for, **287–297**
Pelvis
    ^{11}C-acetate imaging for, 342–343
    ^{18}F-fluorocholine imaging for, 303
    ^{18}F-fluoro-DOPA imaging for, 313–314
    ^{18}F-fluorothymidine imaging for, 335
    ^{18}F-sodium fluoride uptake in, 279–280

PET/CT
- 11C-acetate, **339–344**
- choline, **299–306**
- 18F-fluoride, **277–285, 287–297**
- 18F-fluoro-DOPA, **307–321**
- 18F-fluorothymidine, **331–338**
- for brain, **267–276**
- gallium-69, **323–329**
- standardization of, **259–266**

PET/MRI, radiotracers for, **345–349**
Pheochromocytomas, 308–309, 312–314
Phlogosis, 18F-fluorocholine and, 300
Phospholipid metabolism, in cancer, 346
Phosphorylation, in brain tumors, 300
11C-Pittsburgh Compound B, for brain disorders, 267–268
Pituitary gland tumors
- 11C-acetate imaging for, 340
- 18F-fluorocholine imaging for, 300

11C-PK11195, for brain disorders, 268–269, 274
Plantar fasciitis, 282
Premedication, in 18F-fluoro-DOPA imaging, 309–314
Proliferation imaging, **331–338**. See also Brain tumors; Cancer.
Prostate, cancer of
- 11C-acetate imaging for, 342
- 11C-choline imaging for, 264–265
- 18F-fluorocholine imaging for, 303
- 18F-fluoromethylcholine imaging for, 346

Q

Quantification, of PET/CT, **259–266**
Quantitative Imaging Biomarkers Alliance, 260

R

11C-Raclopride, for brain disorders, 272
Radiological Society of North America, standardized programs of, 260
11C-Radiopharmaceuticals, procedures for, 261
Radiotherapy, 18F-fluorothymidine uptake and, 335–336
Renal osteodystrophy, 293
Rib fractures, 292–294

S

Sacroiliac joint, inflammation of, 280, 290–292
Salivary glands
- 11C-acetate imaging for, 340
- 18F-fluorocholine imaging for, 300

Schizophrenia, 274
Scoliosis, 292
Seizures, 270
Sinusitis, 301
Skull, 18F-sodium fluoride uptake in, 279
Society of Nuclear Medicine and Nuclear Imaging, standardization programs of, 260

18F-Sodium fluoride, **277–285**
- for atherosclerosis detection, 283
- for bone imaging
  - clinical applications of, 288–295
  - for benign conditions, 279–283
  - in pediatric patients, **287–297**
  - normal distribution and, 278–279
  - radiation exposure in, 278
  - technique for, 278, 287–288
  - uptake of, 277–278
- for PET/MRI, 346–347

Somatostatin receptors, gallium-68 labeled. See Gallium-68 labeled somatostatin receptors.
SPECT, for movement disorders, 271–272
Spinal facet arthropathy, 290–291
Spine
- disorders of, 288–292
- 18F-sodium fluoride uptake in, 279–281

Spleen
- accessory, 326
- 11C-acetate imaging for, 341–342
- 18F-fluorocholine imaging for, 302–303

Standardization, of PET/CT, **259–266**
Stomach, cancer of, 335
Striatum, 18F-fluoro-DOPA imaging of, 308, 314–315
Submandibular glands, 18F-fluorocholine imaging for, 300
Sympathetic nervous system, 18F-fluoromisonidazole imaging for, 348

T

Thorax
- 11C-acetate imaging for, 340–341
- 18F-fluorocholine imaging for, 301
- 18F-fluoro-DOPA imaging for, 313
- 18F-fluorothymidine imaging for, 334
- gallium-68 labeled somatostatin receptor imaging for, 327

Thymoma, 301
Thyroid gland
- 11C-acetate imaging for, 340
- 18F-fluorocholine imaging for, 300
- medullary carcinoma of, 18F-fluoro-DOPA imaging for, 308–309, 317–318

Thyroiditis, 18F-fluorocholine for, 301
Total-body scanning, 11C-methionine for, 262
Transitional cell carcinoma, of bladder, 343
Transitional vertebrae, 291–292
Translocator protein, 274

U

Uniform Protocols in Clinical Trials document, 260

V

Vesicular monoamine transporter 2, 271

Moving?

Make sure your subscription moves with you!

To notify us of your new address, find your **Clinics Account Number** (located on your mailing label above your name), and contact customer service at:

Email: journalscustomerservice-usa@elsevier.com

800-654-2452 (subscribers in the U.S. & Canada)
314-447-8871 (subscribers outside of the U.S. & Canada)

Fax number: 314-447-8029

Elsevier Health Sciences Division
Subscription Customer Service
3251 Riverport Lane
Maryland Heights, MO 63043

*To ensure uninterrupted delivery of your subscription, please notify us at least 4 weeks in advance of move.

ELSEVIER